Also by Mary-Ellen Siegel

Her Way

Chemotherapy: Your Weapon Against Cancer
(co-author: Ezra M. Greenspan, M.D.)

What Every Man Should Know About His Prostate
(co-author: Monroe E. Greenberger, M.D.)

Her Way, 2nd edition

More Than a Friend: Dogs with a Purpose
(co-author: Hermine M. Koplin)

REVERSING
HAIR LOSS

Mary-Ellen Siegel, M.S.W.

Senior Teaching Associate
Department of Community Medicine (Social Work)
Mount Sinai School of Medicine, New York

Foreword by
Joel J. Kassimir, M.D.
Clinical Instructor, Department of Dermatology
New York University Medical Center

Illustrations by Lynne Cooper

A Fireside Book
Published by Simon & Schuster, Inc.
New York

All rights reserved including the right of
reproduction in whole or in part in any
form. A Fireside Book, published by Simon
& Schuster, Inc., Simon & Schuster Building, Rockefeller Center, 1230 Avenue of the
Americas, New York, New York 10020.
FIRESIDE and colophon are registered
trademarks of Simon & Schuster, Inc.

Designed by Barbara Marks

Manufactured in the United States of America
Printed by Fairfield Graphics
Bound by Fairfield Graphics

7   9   10   8   6

Library of Congress Cataloging in Publication Data

Siegel, Mary-Ellen.
Reversing hair loss.

"A Fireside book."
Includes index.
1. Baldness—Prevention. 2. Baldness—Treatment.
I. Title.
RL155.S57 1985   616.5′46   85-14373
ISBN 0-671-55469-7

For Walter,
with all my love always

Acknowledgments

I AM MOST GRATEFUL TO THESE HEALTH CARE PROFESSION-als, who were so generous with their time and expertise: Richard Anderson, M.D., Jan AufderHeide, Robert Auerbach, M.D., Arlene Berger, M.S.W., Robert Berger, M.D., Wilma Bergfeld, M.D., Ellyn Bushkin, R.N., M.S., Jack Dalton, M.D., Nancy P. Durr, Ellen Felten, J. Lester Gabrilove, M.D., Michael A. Goldsmith, M.D., Anna Marie Gordon, Ron Gordon, Ph.D., Ezra M. Greenspan, M.D. Richard Hamburg, M.D., Jimmie Holland, M.D., Elliott Jacobs, M.D., Melvin Kahn, M.D. Norman Kanof, M.D., Theodor Kaufman, M.D., Lawrence R. Krakoff, M.D., Stephen Kurtin, M.D., Albert Lafkovits, M.D., Donald Levine, M.D., Carolyn Messner, M.S.W., Phillis Mervis, M.S.W., Edward R. Nida, Norman Orentreich, M.D., Hillard Pearlstein, M.D., Joseph Policar, R.Ph., Michael Reed, M.D., Darrell S. Rigel, M.D., Marcus Ross, R.Ph., John Rothschild, M.D., Ronald Savin, M.D., Edward Settel, M.D., Bernard Simon, M.D., James Storer, M.D., D. Bluford Stough III, M.D., Margot Tallmer, PhD., and Charles Vallis, M.D., Madeline Weiner, R.N.

Joel Kassimer, M.D., was helpful above and beyond all expectations.

I am also grateful to these hair care professionals, who shared their experiences and knowledge with me: Charles Alfieri, David Crespin, Eva Feiger, Francisco of Vidal Sassoon, Edith Imre, Ben Kaplan of Universal Winners, Inc., Hal Z. Laderman of Pantron I, Ray Olsen of Act II, Maurice Mann of Hair Again, Ltd., Evan Miller of Hiar Images, Geroge Roberson, Jerry Roman of Louis Feder/Joseph Fleischer, ken Roper Jr. of Eva Gabor, International, Harvey Russo of Top

Priority, Sy Sperling of Hair Club for Men, Ltd., and the many, many men and women who told me about their feelings and experiences with hair loss and hair restoration.

My particular thanks to the chemotherapy patients who have, for so many years, shared with me their feelings about hair loss.

The helpful staff of the Levy Library at The Mount Sinai School of Medicine always put their hands on what I was looking for. The Medical Arts Department repeatedly came up with just who and what I needed.

Lynne Cooper's contributions were enormous—proving again that Mount Sinai is one big helpful family.

Special thanks to Barbara Wasserman for all her assistance.

The members of my family, with and without hair, have always been an inspiration to me in everything. Thanks for being.

As always, I am grateful for the friendship, help and support received from my colleagues in the Departments of Community Medicine and Social Work at the Mount Sinai School of Medicine.

No book about hair loss, or any other aspect of dermatology, would be complete without a mention of the late Charles Rein, M.D. "Uncle Chuck" was an important figure in my childhood. And even after these many years, his name still opened doors for me in dermatology offices all over New York. I thought of him often, with love, respect and special gratitude, as I interviewed doctors he had trained.

Contents

Foreword

YOU CAN'T FOOL THE GENES...OR CAN YOU? ANY BALD OR balding man will tell you that the reason he lost or is losing his hair is due to his genetic makeup or, put more simply, heredity. Obviously, we can't choose our parents, grand-parents, great-grandparents, or any of the other ancestors whose genes come together in a unique way to produce an individual who may or may not lose his hair. Most of us are genetically predisposed to a variety of medical disorders which sometimes, unfortunately, cannot be cured. As a mat-ter of fact, there are very few diseases that we as physicians can actually cure except infectious diseases. But many prob-lems can be controlled by one therapeutic regime or another.

What about balding? Why have physicians been willing to accept it as an affliction over which they could not exert control? (Not a comfortable feeling for us.) With this attitude, the diabetic might still be without his insulin. But there is one obvious difference between life-threatening illnesses and balding. Balding is not a medical emergency and so doctors have not felt that the benefits justified the risks of experi-mental measures. Despite this, tens of millions of people (many of my colleagues included) have refused to give in without a fight. The fact is that hundreds of millions of dol-lars are spent each year on various over-the-counter prepa-rations and services, such as Biotin, Polysorbate 80, Cystein, herbal astringents, scalp massages, and hair vitamins, with questionable efficacy. These measures are generally supposed to retard hair loss, but it is impossible to measure their effectiveness without testing them scientifically on a representative control group. Only studies of identical twins would tell us whether those who do not use these products lose more hair than those who do.

What has probably inhibited intelligent research on both a clinical and basic science level is the fact that until recently we really did not understand the physiology of male pattern baldness, so randomly rubbing in a variety of lotions or "snake oils" seemed like a senseless way to go about finding a cure.

Imagine our surprise then, when Upjohn's drug minoxidil, approved by the FDA for hypertension in the late 1970s, caused indiscriminate hair growth in almost 90 percent of the high blood pressure patients who took it internally. This stimulated extensive serious work to determine whether minoxidil applied topically to the head might prove to be the ultimate remedy for baldness. These continuing studies have shown interesting and positive results.

In the meantime, it is now becoming clear that the cause of balding is not the male hormone testosterone (if it were, *all* men would be bald), but the capability of the hair follicles to produce the enzyme 5 alpha reductase which converts testosterone into another hormone, dihydrotestosterone.

That's the basis of a hair transplant. Ever wonder why the hairs on the sides of the head—the "fringe"—don't fall out? They are incapable of producing 5 alpha reductase. Therefore, dermatologists and plastic surgeons can move these follicles surgically and transplant them to the top of the head. There they will grow as they were genetically coded just as they did in their original location. The hairs don't know that they have been moved. You could even put them on the tip of your nose and the graft would take.

I'm sure that the twenty-eight clinical investigators now studying minoxidil in university centers across the country would agree that it is not a panacea, but the first breakthrough, which has been demonstrated in closely scrutinized, scientifically conducted double-blind studies to be the best we have in 1985. Upjohn is now working on improved methods of application of minoxidil, which would increase its effectiveness in a greater percentage of patients, and on a second-generation drug with greater potency. Competing products from other companies can't be far behind. The next few years should prove to be very exciting.

Joel J. Kassimir, M.D.
Clinical Instructor
Department of Dermatology
New York University Medical Center

Introduction

FOR MANY YEARS PHYSICIANS TOLD US NOT TO WASTE OUR MONEY on worthless concoctions to cure baldness that is caused by common "pattern baldness." But now excitement pervades the offices of dermatologists in big university centers as well as in small towns.

Why?

A new drug, called minoxidil, is actually growing hair on balding heads. So after many years of skeptical shrugs by scientists and physicians, a treatment has been developed that demonstrates obvious value. Doctors no longer tell patients they have nothing to offer: they are writing prescriptions for minoxidil. Pharmacists, marveling at the results, are working overtime to fill the prescriptions.

The official Upjohn investigators who have been studying minoxidil have found the drug to be safe and very effective. They generally are excited enough about the results to use the drug on their own private patients, their balding relatives, and themselves. And at medical meetings across the country they share their exciting findings with other physicians.

But minoxidil isn't the *only* development in the quest to reverse baldness. Dermatologists and plastic surgeons can now perform hair transplants, usually in a doctor's office, that far surpass the earliest procedures. Today, men, women, and children who never thought it possible have hair again.

Other people, whose hair loss is profound, or who want

the full head of their youth, are finding that the new hair pieces or hair weaves are so natural, no one but their hair stylist knows for sure. Good care at home and in a salon can do much to alleviate hair loss.

Today, nobody has to *look* bald anymore. Many people don't even have to *be* bald anymore. And certainly they need not look foolish or phony if they choose to compensate for hair loss by the use of modern technology.

You don't have to hide your head under a wardrobe of hats. Nor do you have to add some shine to your bald head and declare "bald is better," unless you really mean it. Too many people utter those words just because they don't know what they can do about their baldness. Fear, ignorance, naivete, disbelief, or despair are no longer excuses.

In the pages that follow, we will tell you the whole story about minoxidil, transplants, and all the other excellent new ways to reverse your hair loss—how to grow it back, how to put it back, and how you can make what you *do* have look its best.

Mary-Ellen Siegel, M.S.W.
Senior Teaching Associate
Department of Community Medicine
  (Social Work)
Mount Sinai School of Medicine, New York

Going Bald:
Who, How and Why

CHAPTER 1

The Most Common Cause of Hair Loss: Pattern Baldness

ONE DAY WHEN MICHIGAN STATE SOPHOMORE TED LANSING (not his real name) was shaving, he noticed his hair was thinning. He looked again and realized it wasn't thinning all over, just around the temples. His father still had a full head of hair. So did his older brother. "How could my hair be receding?" Ted wondered.

Only a year or two ago Ted had suffered through pimples and oily hair. Now he had this new problem with which to contend. So, when he came home for Christmas vacation, he went to see the dermatologist who had taken care of his adolescent acne.

The doctor took a good look, and shook his head. "Ted," he said, "this isn't something we can clear up like the acne."

"Why not?" Ted asked.

The dermatologist explained that, young as Ted was, he appeared to be suffering from a case of "garden variety" male pattern baldness, or MPB. Sometimes described as common baldness, it accounts for 95 percent of all baldness. It strikes women as well as men, and can start at any time after puberty.

Ted's dermatologist had no trouble making the diagnosis. He looked carefully at Ted's scalp, noticing that the hair was thinning around the temples and on the crown. Looking at Ted's hair through a thick magnifying glass, and examining a few strands under a microscope in order to determine the ratio of growing-shedding hairs, the doctor noted that there were two distinct kinds of hair on Ted's scalp. One was of normal coarseness, but the other had a thinner shaft. He began to question Ted about his family, and Ted recalled that in the family photograph album there were a number of pictures of his maternal grandfather, taken during summer vacations, in all of which Grandpa wore a hat.

"To cover his bald head, I bet," Ted exclaimed.

The Three Crucial Factors in Balding

Ted's doctor also explained that men who bald young have often had trouble with acne during their teens. A capricious, rather than an excessive portion of androgens (the collective term for a group of male sex hormones) causes both situations. Although studies do not support the commonly believed theory that bald men have a higher androgen level in their blood, the correlation of androgens, acne, excessive hair on the chest, ability to grow a full beard and baldness has long been noticed. Three factors—androgens, age, and heredity—are needed for male pattern baldness like Ted's to take place; although the precise proportions and amounts required remain an enigma.

Who Becomes Bald?

Who actually suffers hair loss? Most men, it seems. Twelve percent of men aged twenty-five show some signs of loss, forty percent of all men in their thirties suffer noticeable hair loss, and half of all men in their forties have lost a great deal of hair. A whopping seventy percent of men over sixty-five have a significant loss of hair.

We are all potentially susceptible to baldness. From puberty men and women have androgens circulating in their body, although men have more than women. Estrogens (female hormones) in women counteract some of the effects of androgen.

A great number of us, men and women, inherit the genes that can lead to baldness as we age. If Ted's father had been bald, Ted would have had a fifty percent chance of inheriting the gene. If his mother had also carried the gene—even if it hadn't shown up yet—baldness would have been Ted's expected legacy.

Often, the color and quality of your hair is inherited from some relative. If that relative is balding, you may inherit that propensity too.

Is It Your Genes?

You probably learned about genetics in your high school biology course, but even if you remember the Mendelian principles and definitions of autosomal dominance, autosomal recessive, monohybrid inheritance, variable penetrance and variable expressivity you will also need a crystal ball. Based on genetics alone, no one has yet been able to predict with any precision who will bald and who won't.

Many dermatologists tell puzzling stories of identical twins: one of whom balded while the other didn't. Theoretically, their genetic programming and body chemistry (including androgens) were identical. So why did baldness show up in one twin and not the other? No one has yet come up with a definitive explanation, but some doctors suggest an environmental factor may be at work.

Less confusing, but still puzzling, are the instances where brothers differ in their balding process, sons bald when fathers don't, and mothers with full heads of hair have daughters who don't.

Since baldness is so common, it's difficult to find a family without a few bald members. If there is baldness on *both* sides of your family, it's hard to escape the inevitable, and it is a good guess you will start the balding process at an early age.

Defying Your Genes

For baldness to occur, genes are important, but the presence of sufficient androgens is also crucial. There have been documented cases in which one identical twin's testicles were damaged or removed before puberty, resulting in castration.

As he grew older he retained a nice full head of hair. The twin who was not castrated gradually lost his hair in a typical MPB fashion. Years later, the castrated twin received injections of male hormones and promptly began to lose hair. Within six months he was as bald as his brother.

You can't choose your ancestors, and you can't stop the clock. But, as noted above, one *can* avoid most of the androgens. How? Castration. That's one sure way to avoid baldness. If you look at old paintings of eunuchs in harems, you will notice they always have beautiful heads of hair. But that's a high price to pay just to keep a headful of hair, isn't it?

Both hormonal castration (receiving substantial doses of female hormones) and surgical castration (removal of both testicles and, if past puberty, the addition of female hormones) can stop male pattern baldness. Many transsexuals have found this out. Prior to the surgery that changed her from male to female, Dr. Renee Richards, the well-known ophthalmologist and tennis coach, underwent hormonal castration. She says, "Female hormones do some marvelous and radical things. They make you grow breasts, they shrink your testicles, they change the outline of your body, and they'll even stop you from going bald."

Perhaps it worked for Dr. Richards, but there's no guarantee that baldness will completely cease. The adrenal glands also produce androgens. In any case, hair that has been lost is unlikely to grow back. Other feminizing effects of any form of castration, some of which Dr. Richards describes, include reduced musculature and increased fat deposition, hot flashes, and loss of ability to have and maintain an erection. There's no need to continue with the list; it's obvious why no one would opt for castration *just* to avoid hair loss.

Those transsexuals who have changed from female to male find that if their genetic code reads "baldness," the addition of androgens signals the baldness to take place.

If one is cursed with the ineluctable alliance of that mischievous trio—genes, androgens, and age, how can hair loss ever be reversed? To answer that question, it is first necessary to know a little about how hair grows.

How Hair Grows

The root of each hair grows in a follicle, which is formed before birth and nourished by blood-bearing capillaries beneath the scalp. The follicles themselves are little pouchlike depressions which line the pores in the skin (on your scalp, arms, chest, etc.).

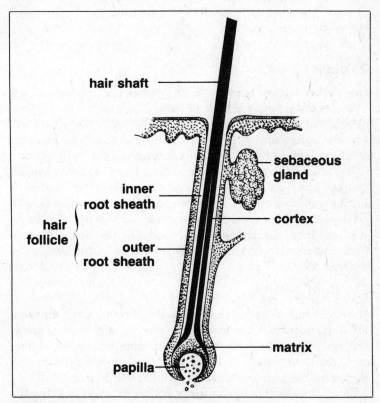

A Single Hair
The visible hair is the end-product of the hair matrix, which grows from deep inside the follicle. The papilla, at the base of the hair, is the root which receives needed nutrients from the follicle. The visible hair shaft is covered by a cuticle, which acts as a protective shield. Beneath the cuticle is the cortex, which makes up most of the hair's bulk.

Genetics play a role in determining the shape of the follicles, and that shape determines whether a person will have straight or curly hair. This explains why certain families, races and nationality groups have characteristic types of hair.

Apart from heredity, hair growth depends on the follicles receiving a normal amount of blood supply, oxygen, nutrients, growth and thyroid hormones (and in some areas of the body, sex hormones). A lack of any of these can diminish or even prevent hair growth. The hair itself can be damaged by strong chemicals.

Types of Hair

Human babies are born with *lanugo* hair, a very fine, sometimes colorless hair which is shed after birth. The downy, almost invisible hair that covers most of an adult's body (except palms and soles), and often covers a bald person's scalp, is lanugo hair. It is usually referred to a *vellus* hair.

Vellus hair later becomes *terminal* hair, which is longer, coarser and has a specific color. At puberty, the male sex hormones (androgens) cause the vellus hair on the face of adolescent males to become terminal hair. If not shaved, it will produce a mustache and beard. On the heads of both men and women, terminal hair coarsens still further.

Cycle of Growth

Hair growth is not continuous. Each follicle has its own timetable. At any one time some hairs on the head may be growing, other hairs may be resting, and some may be shedding.

The growing stage is called the *anagen* phase. About 85–90 percent of a person's hair is always in this phase—during which the cells in each hair root actively divide, making the hair grow longer.

At the conclusion of the growing stage, hair goes into the *telogen* stage. Approximately ten to fifteen percent of hair is always at this phase, during which the hair root rests. When this happens, cells stop dividing and the hair stops growing. It separates from the root and begins to shed. This resting and shedding phase lasts from two to six months. Telogen hairs, when pushed out by a new hair growing up from below, appear on combs and brushes, in the sink or shower, and on your new blue suit. Ideally, the hairs are replaced as fast as they are lost, and although brushing or washing may hasten the fallout, the loss would probably occur anyway within a few days.

The loss of this ten to fifteen percent is unimportant, since the average adult has approximately 100,000 hairs, which shed in random fashion. Blondes have slightly more but thinner hairs; redheads have larger but somewhat fewer follicles, and thus thicker hair. The rate and duration of hair growth varies with the individual.

Amount of Growth and Loss

On the scalp, hair grows at an average of about one-half to one inch a month, and there is really no way anyone can make their hair grow faster than it is programmed to.

Daily hair loss can vary, but the average person loses upwards of one hundred hairs a day from scattered areas of the head.

Normally, hair grows back at the same rate at which it is lost, although there are times when this cycle is altered. In the next chapter we will discuss some of these conditions. However, most abnormal hair loss, or *alopecia*, as physicians call it, is due to common pattern baldness.

How Do the Three Crucial Factors Work Together?

While we know the factors—androgens, genetics and age— which come together to do their mischief, *how* do they do it? The precise answer is still unknown, but on some matters there is agreement among the medical experts.

Pattern baldness can begin as early as puberty, with the secretion of androgens. That is when boys' and most girls' straight frontal hairlines change to an M-shaped hairline, sometimes known as a widow's peak. This occurs because some of the follicles miniaturize, or shrink. This change in hairline is *not* necessarily a precursor to balding. But if the miniaturization continues and extends, terminal hair will become vellus hair and finally disappear, resulting in loss of the hair on other parts of the scalp. Some people lose hair only at the forehead; the crown stays intact for a long time. Others initially lose only the hair on the crown. Those men who are destined to early baldness usually lose it in both places. Eventually, in the truly bald, the two areas meet, and the only remaining hair is at the base and sides of the head. Because those follicles are not genetically coded to miniaturize, the familiar horseshoe pattern of sideburns and fringe remains indefinitely. Men you see without it have either shaved it off (à la Yul Brynner and Telly Savalas) or have lost their hair from another cause, such as chemotherapy.

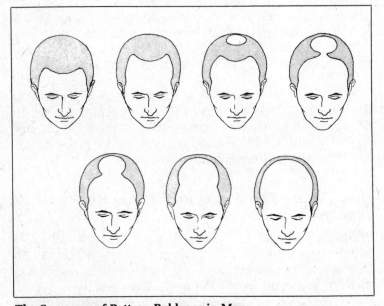

The Sequence of Pattern Baldness in Men
Some men begin to lose hair at the hairline; for others hair loss begins on the crown; still others lose both simultaneously. Eventually, the two bald areas meet, and all that remains is a horsehoe fringe.

The Real Culprits: 5 Alpha Reductase and DHT

Those male hormones that at puberty make hair coarser, also cause the growth of pubic hair, underarm hair, and on men, hair on the ears, nostrils, chin, chest, arms and legs.

Some of this new hair growth is caused by a male hormone called testosterone, but some of it is caused by an even more powerful hormone, dihydrotestosterone (DHT). A catalyzing enzyme, 5 alpha reductase, transforms or metabolizes testosterone into its derivative, DHT.

This same DHT "taketh as well as giveth." In certain target follicles, the hair hungrily grabs DHT, which unfortunately makes the follicles miniaturize. As the hair follicles grow smaller, the hair growing cycles become progressively shorter and/or the resting periods become longer. This causes the hairs to get thinner and shorter, and less deeply placed in the follicle.

This process, which describes typical male pattern baldness, is not always immediately apparent. Hair may be lost at a normal rate, but the regrowth is a finer, thinner, even babylike hair. Eventually, there is no regrowth.

Because the receptor cells in the hair follicles vary on different parts of the head and body, DHT can make hair grow in some areas and cease to grow in others. Paradoxically, this occurs simultaneously. Even while a man is balding, hair growth may increase on his chest, back and limbs.

Some studies show that hairs taken from the frontal region of a balding person's scalp have a higher level of DHT than hairs from the same area in a nonbalding scalp, but these studies are not fully confirmed. Many experts believe the real culprit is the enzyme 5 alpha reductase. If that enzyme could be harnessed and kept at a distance, they feel, hair would not be unhappily influenced by DHT. In their view, as long as DHT is allowed to go unchecked, the genetically programmed scalp will continue to bald.

Individual Time Clock

When does this balding occur? Why does it happen to some men as early as their mid-teens, others not until their forties, and still others not until their sixties or later? Here too, genetics plays a part. Men (and women) inherit a time clock that determines where, when, and if they will begin to lose their hair. In some, the time clock seems to click away at full speed, but in others the process may begin so slowly that for many years it is barely discernible.

At this writing, my twenty-seven-year-old son appears to have a full head of hair. One day recently he called me and said, "Mom, remember that time when I was six and I cut my head while I was playing hide and seek? And I had to have stitches?"

"Sure I remember," I replied. "The doctor said there would be a scar, but your hairline covers it."

"Well, it doesn't anymore," he said.

I tell this anecdote to illustrate the fact that while hair loss occurs to some extent in most men, it can be very gradual. Without his scar as a marker, I'll wager Peter wouldn't have noticed his scalp's time clock had begun to tick.

Problems Specific to Women

Numerous women also suffer from pattern baldness, but they don't like to talk about it, so many people are unaware of its prevalence.

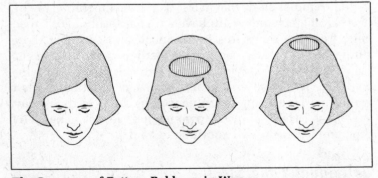

The Sequence of Pattern Baldness in Women
Women's pattern baldness usually consists of thinning rather than true baldness. Their pattern is similar to men's: loss may begin at the hairline or crown, or occur simultaneously in both areas.

The causes of pattern baldness in women are the same as in men. Androgens also circulate in womens' bodies, produced by both the adrenal glands and the ovaries. While female hormones—estrogens—counteract some of the effects, including hair loss, the androgens are often powerful enough to do exactly what they do in men: miniaturize those follicles whose genetic markers read "bald." The condition can occur in young women, but it is more likely after surgical or natural menopause, when estrogen levels decrease.

In the event of some endocrine disorder, (to be discussed in chapter two) a women may produce more than the normal amount of male hormones. This can trigger baldness, as well as other masculinizing effects. These are, however, correctible with treatment. If she is taking androgenic-dominant oral contraceptives, she may suffer hair loss resembling MPB.

Frequently this baldness is not reversible by simple means. She may take some comfort in knowing her hair loss is more subtle than that of the men in her life, but she will have good reason to be upset.

Women who are genetically programmed to lose their hair often also suffer a paradox similar to that of the bald man who develops a hairy chest. While her scalp hair thins, she grows some facial and body hair. Like the baldness itself, this effect tends to be subtle. If excessive it may be due to an endocrine disorder. In that case, it should be brought to the attention of a physician.

Not all hair loss is due to pattern baldness, and in the next chapter we discuss some other causes and what you can do about them. But ninety-five percent of hair loss *is* caused by pattern baldness, which depends on the three factors: androgens (DHT, to be precise), genetics and age. All are needed to produce a bald head. While some people will escape almost indefinitely the ravages of hair loss, others will not be so lucky.

But don't give up—reversing hair loss is no longer an impossibility. Many men (and women too) have been part of the Upjohn study involving a drug called minoxidil (see chapter 5), or have received the drug from their doctor, and have astounded friends with new hair growth. Others have sought some of the surgical or cosmetic methods that seem to be improving day by day. No man or woman has to *look* bald, and in many instances, they don't even have to *be* bald. In sections Two, Three, Four, and Six we will delve into the ways in which hair loss can be slowed, reversed or camouflaged.

CHAPTER 2

Other Causes,
Temporary and Permanent

ONE OF MY EARLIEST MEMORIES CONCERNS HAIR LOSS. JUST BE-
fore I was three years old I had scarlet fever. A few months
following the illness, my hair began to fall out. With my
blond stringy strands of hair I was a rather pathetic-looking
sight. Then my parents gave me a short haircut, and I thought
I looked just fine.

It was December, and one day in our local five and dime,
Santa Claus was giving out little gifts to every child whose
parent bought a ticket. No one had yet invented the concept
of nonsexist toys and so Santa gave guns to all the boys and
dolls to all the girls. When Santa handed me a gun I was
crestfallen. Santa, whom I thought knew everything, obviously thought I was a boy. It was quickly straightened out,
but I was humiliated by the implications of my recent hair
loss, and I cried all the way home.

The spring after I turned thirteen I developed pneumonia
accompanied by a high fever. Just as I was about to begin
high school my hair began to fall out. My parents hauled me
off to a dermatologist, who recommended some lotions and
gave me heat lamp treatments. Again I had a short haircut
but, mercifully, this time no one thought I was a boy. Nonetheless, I was so dreadfully self-conscious I wouldn't go out
without a hat. The hair eventually grew back, just as it would
have without any treatment. Meanwhile, I drew some con-

solation from the knowledge that at least people were trying to do something about it.

My experience was not unique. Illnesses, accompanied by high fevers such as I had, severe infections, and various metabolic changes, can cause temporary hair loss sometimes two or three months after the illness.

Although only a small percentage of temporary or permanent hair loss is due to causes other than pattern baldness, each is devastating to the man, woman or child who suffers from one of them.

Telogen Effluvium

Here's what happened in my episodes of hair loss and in similar situations which may have happened to you. The ten to fifteen percent of your telogen (or resting) hairs that were destined to come out are doing so at a greater rate than normal. Instead of shedding up to 100 hairs a day, you're losing up to 700 a day. This is called *telogen effluvium*: excessive hair loss during the resting stage. You will remember that on page 24 we explained that ten to fifteen percent of your hair is usually in the telogen stage. In telogen effluvium this percentage increases to 30, or sometimes to 50 percent. The other 50 to 70 percent of your hair continues to grow, and it is just a matter of time before the hair growth cycle resumes its usual pattern.

In other instances, hair may shed at its usual rate, but fail to grow.

If you notice excessive hair on your brush or pillow, or if your hair looks thinner than usual, you should think about the following possibilities.

Am I Losing Much Hair?

You can do a simple test that physicians use to discover if hair shedding is excessive. With your thumb and index finger grasp fifteen to twenty hairs near the scalp and pull them slowly but firmly. Normally two or three hairs will come out. But if six or more hairs come out, it is a sign of trouble! And, of course, if you feel that more than the usual amount of hair is coming out, or if your head looks sparser than before, do some self-evaluation even before you seek professional help.

Look at the tips of the hairs that have been shed. Pointed or tapered ends indicate the hair has come out by the roots. Jagged or broken ends are the result of breakage.

Traction Alopecia

Have you been wearing tight ponytails, braids or cornrows? Using tight barrettes, curlers, hair pins or even styling combs? This can cause *traction alopecia*, a condition in which hair that has been pulled too tightly begins to fall out and, in some instances, doesn't grow back.

This is what happened to Gail. She was a devoted reader of fashion magazines, and she loved to try new hairstyles. Her wonderful high cheekbones and almond-shaped eyes were set off by the little cornrows she liked to wear. To achieve the look she liked, Gail enlisted her friend, Pauline, to help her pull the hair as tightly as possible. One day Pauline exclaimed, "Gail, you actually have spaces in the back where the hair has come out."

Gail was horrified. Although the damage wasn't extensive, it had injured the follicles and led to permanent loss. If her hair had merely broken off at the shaft, it would have re-grown. As long as the follicles have not been damaged, traction alopecia can easily be reversed merely by stopping the traction.

Friction Alopecia

Jim wouldn't budge without his cap. He wore it all day long, and would have worn it to bed if his mother hadn't been firmly opposed. One day she noticed his hair was thinning just in the area where the hat fit most snugly.

Jim was suffering from *friction alopecia*, a condition that develops from constantly wearing a hat, a wig, or some other close-fitting head covering, or from rubbing one's head on a pillow. His hair was broken off so close to the scalp it looked as if it had come out by the roots.

When Jim finally agreed to give up the hat for most of the day, his hair began to grow back.

Physical Stress

Before panicking about hair loss, think about any shocks or stresses to your body (like severe infections, high fevers or the flu) you may have undergone recently. Like myself, some people are vulnerable to stress-induced hair shedding. The trauma causes an unusual number of their hairs to go into the telogen phase, and two or three months later shedding begins. Even emotional stress can cause hair loss, but that is rare.

Diet Deficiencies

Peggy looked great. She finally went on the diet she had talked about for years. "No doctors, no Weight Watchers, no pills, just will-power," Peggy boasted. "I just stopped eat-ing—almost," she declared. Peggy's figure looked beautiful, but her hair certainly didn't. It began to fall out faster than she shed those pounds.

What went wrong? Peggy didn't know that hair follicles require protein to function normally, and so a crash diet, or even a well-planned weight loss, can lead to hair loss for some people. A vegetarian diet lacking in protein can also cause hair to fall out. Hair follicles are low on the priority list of places the body sends protein, so if there isn't enough to go around, the hair suffers. When sufficient protein is added to the diet, hair loss will stop. Zinc deficiency can also lead to hair loss. However, adding extra protein or zinc to an otherwise normal diet will not result in more or better hair growth.

On the advice of her doctor, Peggy went to a nutritionist who helped her plan a good maintenance diet, sufficient in protein to allow for regrowth of her hair, but not her waist-line.

Pregnancy

I began researching this book just at the time my daughter gave birth to her second child. When Josh was about three months old, Betsy called me one morning and asked if I had read up on hair loss following pregnancy. She said her brush was uncharacteristically filled with hair.

"That didn't happen after Matthew was born," she said.

I was able to reassure her that many women report some hair loss three or four months after they have a baby. There are individual differences, and it may happen after one pregnancy but not another.

Here's what happens: the hormonal effects of pregnancy *lessen* the usual shedding rate. To compensate, more of the hair follicles go into the resting phase after the baby is born, causing increasing hair shedding. However, hair growth eventually makes up for the hair loss, so I was glad to assure Betsy that she'll have as much hair as ever at Josh's first birthday party.

The Pill

Women who have stopped taking "the pill" often report that they are losing hair in much the same way as new mothers. Women who are predisposed to androgenic pattern baldness may experience hair loss while they are taking androgenic-dominant oral contraceptives. If this happens to you, speak with your doctor about changing to an estrogen-dominant pill. Don't switch without discussing it with your gynecologist or family physician: estrogen-dominant contraception is not for every woman.

Drug-Caused Hair Loss

Certain drugs that may cause hair loss include some, but not all, medications for hypertension, cardiac conditions, gout, arthritis, thyroidism, acne, nausea, psychiatric disorders, and some anticoagulants (blood thinners), anticonvulsants, amphetamines, antibiotics, and hormones. Elevated levels of Vitamin A can cause hair loss. Many people take high doses of Vitamin A without a doctor's advice, only to discover this unhappy consequence. Because kidney dialysis patients often develop high levels of Vitamin A, they may suffer hair loss. Cancer chemotherapy drugs can also cause sudden and extreme hair loss; that will be discussed in chapter ten.

A word of caution: do not decide to discontinue a drug that has been prescribed for you because you think it is causing hair loss. Instead, speak with the physician who prescribed it to learn if hair loss is a possibility. If so, ask if another drug can be substituted.

Chemical Damage to Hair

My friend Cynthia, in anticipation of a long-awaited vacation in the Caribbean, spent a day at a local beauty parlor. She had her mousy brown hair stripped of color, then dyed a lovely shade of blond. She had always wanted curls, so she also had a permanent. Then she went on her vacation— where she enjoyed sunny ocean breezes, surfing, and diving into the chlorine pool. Before her vacation was over Cynthia's hair was a mess, and she spent the last few days of her vacation hiding it under a turban.

The chemicals used in bleaching, dyeing, or permanent waving, if used improperly, can cause serious damage. When one or more of these treatments is done on the same day, the combined effects can cause hair to break off close to the scalp. Too much sunshine, brushing, hot irons for straightening or curling, or "teasing" can also cause hair to break. Cynthia had abused her hair, but fortunately the damage was only temporary. If her scalp had been injured there might have been follicular destruction, and her hair would not have grown back.

Consultation with a Physician

If you think you know the cause of your hair loss, you may want to give it a fair chance to correct itself. But if you don't see prompt improvement, consult a physician. Your physician is the person who can best evaluate the causes of hair loss and determine what and if something should be done about it. Your corner health food store proprietor, barber, beautician or a staffer at a non-medical so-called hair clinic, are not the first people to consult when you experience hair loss.

What kind of physician should you see? Many people initially see their general family physician or a specialist in internal medicine. A general physician who knows you well may be able to readily recognize the cause. In some instances, hair loss may be the first symptom of a medical problem that should be treated. If not, your family doctor may refer you to a dermatologist, an expert in disorders of the skin and hair. You can, of course, go directly to a dermatologist. A well-trained dermatologist has a firm background in medicine and can do many of the required medical tests, or can send you to an internist, if that is indicated.

If you are a man, and the hair loss appears to be typical male pattern baldness, the physician may suggest some of the methods we will discuss in sections Two, Three and Four.

The physician will ask you a number of questions about your family history, and when the trouble first began. S/he will discuss with you the possibility that your hair loss is caused by traction, friction, chemical damage, physical stress, diet deficiencies, or pregnancy; as well as by any medicines you have been taking regularly or occasionally. If none of these are the cause, the physician will evaluate you for endocrine or other medical problems.

Endocrine and Other Medical Disorders

Some endocrine disorders can cause hair loss, and if the dermatologist suspects a woman is suffering from this, he or she will check for signs of infertility and virilization, and order a plasma testosterone level test. An elevated level indicates a need to see a gynecologist or endocrinologist for a more complete evaluation.

Connective tissue diseases such as systemic lupus erythematosus, rheumatoid arthritis and various chronic illnesses can all cause hair loss.

When the cause of the hair loss is not readily apparent, the doctor will perform a microscopic examination of the patient's hair, and various blood tests. Iron deficiency anemia and secondary syphilis, as well as endocrine disorders such as overactive or underactive thyroidism, polycystic ovaries and diabetes, sometimes cause hair loss.

A correction, where possible, of the underlying condition will stop the hair loss and allow for regrowth. If hair loss is caused by a medication or drug, eliminating the drug (or switching to others) will solve the problem.

While hair loss is terribly upsetting when it occurs, most of the time the problems only last one to six months, and will usually clear up spontaneously or with medical advice. But some hair loss problems are difficult to treat.

Alopecia Areata

About one quarter of a million people suffer from *alopecia areata*, a truly confusing and upsetting condition, in which hair comes out by the roots and stubbornly refuses to grow back. It is the second most common form of hair loss after pattern baldness. It strikes children and young adults with more frequency than older people, but can affect anyone. It usually appears first as one or more small, round or oval, smooth patches on the head or beard—varying in size from that of a penny, to a diameter of more than two inches. It may come on suddenly, without any other symptoms. In alopecia areata, the affected hair follicles slow down their production for months or even years, remaining alive below the surface, but growing no visible hair above the skin.

In milder cases of alopecia areata only a few of these patches develop, and with or without treatment the hair regenerates within a year. But in some unlucky people the condition persists and continues to spread, and eventually they lose all their hair. This condition is called alopecia totalis or alopecia universalis.

At the present time, no one knows with any certainty the cause of alopecia areata. Experts believe it is an immuno-

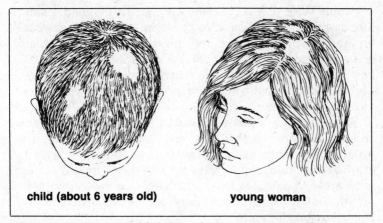

child (about 6 years old)   young woman

Alopecia Areata in Child (left) and Young Woman (right)
Alopecia areata usually begins with hair loss in patchy areas on the
scalp.

logical or autoimmune condition in which the body forms
antibodies against some of the hair follicles. Researchers believe that heredity may play a role in its development because
allergic or autoimmune conditions, as well as alopecia areata,
often appear in more than one family member.

Like many illnesses which depend on an altered immune
system, alopecia areata may follow severe emotional stress
or trauma. Physicians from the University of Padua in Italy
noted that 87.5 percent of the forty-eight alopecia areata patients they studied had experienced a stressful life event
within six months of the disease's appearance. A majority of
the patients had suffered a very serious loss, such as the
death or departure of a close friend or family member.

Children who have suffered a severe loss, such as a parent's death or divorce, will sometimes develop the condition.
However, it is not a psychiatric or emotional disorder, nor
is it caused by ordinary, everyday stress. The loss of hair and
the uncertainty about regrowth do play havoc with mental
health, but psychotherapeutic intervention will not cure the
problem.

People with alopecia areata are usually in good general health and are often reassured to learn that hair grows back on most people. Unfortunately, physicians cannot with any certainty assure a patient *when* and *if* this will occur. The fact that the hair follicles are still alive, even if temporarily dormant, supports the old saying, "Where there's life, there's hope."

There is no cure that will turn off the condition, but successful treatment at this time can "signal" the follicles to produce hair again. Each of these treatments has a downside. For instance, monthly injections of cortisone in and around mild areas of patching can cause new hair growth within a month, but do not prevent new patches from developing elsewhere on the scalp.

A tarlike synthetic substance called anthralin is another treatment which can produce hair growth in six to eight weeks, but the substance is very irritating to the skin and, like cortisone, does not prevent new patches from developing elsewhere.

Extensive alopecia areata and alopecia totalis are very difficult to treat. Cortisone is far more effective when given orally than it is when injected into the site of the problem, so it is sometimes prescribed for this condition. However, there are adverse side effects to long-term cortisone therapy, and when patients stop the drug, the hair may also stop growing.

Some medical centers and dermatologists apply strong chemicals called dinitrochlorobenzene (DNCB) and squaric acid dibutyl ester to the affected area. These chemicals produce an allergic reaction, which looks and feels like poison oak or poison ivy. The skin becomes inflamed, halting the continued process of alopecia areata, and allowing for regrowth. The treatment is continued until, finally, the follicles are signaled to resume activity and treatment is no longer needed.

Another new and effective treatment for extensive alopecia areata is called PUVA, in which a light sensitizing medication (psoralen) is applied topically (to the surface of the affected area) or taken internally. The patient is then exposed to ultraviolet light (UVA). The long-range effects of intense ultraviolet light on the skin are still unknown, and because this treatment must be given a few times a week for several months, it is time consuming and not without some risk.

British physicians reported an interesting case in 1982. Two women who had suffered from long-standing cases of total hair loss from alopecia areata responded to the new drug, minoxidil, with significant hair growth. The drug has achieved some measure of success when applied to the scalp of other patients suffering from alopecia areata. Minoxidil is discussed in depth in chapter 5.

For many patients however, the only way to avoid the unhappy look of bare, patchy areas, at least until hair grows back, is to wear a hairpiece or wig. More about that in chapters 8 and 9. On the horizon are drugs to regulate the immune response, and newer treatments which signal the hair follicles to begin production.

Congenital Alopecia

Although somewhat rare, *congenital alopecia* may result in bare spots, sparse coverage, or complete baldness. Abnormalities of teeth, skin or nails may also be present. Children born with this condition are unlikely to develop hair later.

Seborrhea Capitis

Many dermatologists say that this is the single most common cause of hair loss in women. People with this condition have perpetually oily scalps and hair, excessively thick dandruff scales and crust, along with soreness and itching. Their front hair is sparse, and tends to fall out when combed. Although androgens are a contributing cause, they are not the sole cause. A low-fat diet can help reduce the secretion of sebum, the thick, fatty, semifluid of the sebaceous glands. Special attention to cleanliness, adequate amounts of vitamin B complex, and topical use of steroids may also be helpful. Some dermatologists recommend massage for this condition (although not for most other forms of hair loss); many feel that stress may exacerbate the problem.

Congenital and Inherited Abnormalities

Some hair shaft structural abnormalities, in which the hair is so fragile that it breaks off close to the root, leave the person with little or no hair. In some instances hair is strawlike, unmanageable, and very sparse. All the hair may be involved, or the condition may be patchy. These hair abnormalities result from defects of the hair shaft and the root, and may be linked with metabolic disturbances. Some of these conditions improve at puberty or, in women, during pregnancy or when taking oral contraceptives. Medical treatment is not very successful for most genetic conditions, however. Cosmetic replacement of hair is generally the most satisfactory plan.

Infections

Tinea Capitis, more commonly know as ringworm, is a fungus infection more frequently found in children than adults. It is an infection of the hair and scalp, and can cause patchy, scaly, noninflammatory areas on the scalp from which hairs break off. In another type of this fungus, there is a small, elevated, inflammatory pus-filled mass, devoid of hair. These infections respond well to medication, resulting in hair regrowth.

Some local infections, serious viruses and bacterial infections can destroy the follicles, or leave scar tissue, resulting in the failure of hair to regrow.

Trichotillomania

Trichotillomania is a compulsion, usually unconscious, to pull or tear out one's hair. It will often result in patchy or diffuse alopecia. It is more common in children and the elderly, but has been seen in all age groups. Some children and adults do not realize they have pulled out their hair, so when they seek medical care, trichotillomania is often misdiagnosed as alopecia areata. In preschool children this behavior is analogous to thumb sucking or nail biting, and usually does not represent serious psychological problems. Older children and adults are likely to need psychotherapeutic intervention. Most often, hair will grow back when it is no longer being pulled out.

Moles and Cancers

Little or no hair will grow from a mole on the head, but if the mole is removed, and no scar tissue remains, hair will begin to grow. A patch of alopecia may result from the removal of some growths or cancers.

Cicatrical Alopecia

Cicatrical alopecias, or "burned-out" areas can develop from any medical or physical assault to the head, as well as from an accident, infection or burn. Damage done in the name of beauty treatments as described on page 36, can also result in permanent damage. Hair may not grow back on the resultant scar tissue.

Senescent Alopecia

Diffuse thinning often occurs in men and women over the age of fifty, and increases in the sixties and seventies. The condition in women can be helped by estrogen, topically applied to the head.

Anagen Effluvium

When extensive hair loss occurs within several days, it is usually attributed to anagen arrest or anagen effluvium. A metabolic catastrophy, poisoning, cancer chemotherapy drugs, radiation or acute starvation, can arrest the growth of the hair root and cause hairs to break off at the rate of hundreds, or even thousands a day.

The effect is startling to both the patient and others, even though the hair loss may be expected. In most instances, hair will grow back when the cause of the hair loss is removed. Hair regrows after chemotherapy drugs are discontinued, and often in between treatments. In chapter 10, we discuss hair loss from chemotherapy in greater depth.

Other Causes

Even for a highly experienced dermatologist or other medical specialist (such as an endocrinologist), hair loss can remain a mystery. Using a magnifying glass, a dermatologist can often judge if a follicle is alive, if it has the potential for regrowth. If in doubt, doctors will on occasion do a biopsy of the scalp to obtain a diagnosis, and to determine if the follicles are alive.

However, regardless of the cause of hair loss there is still hope. If hair cannot be grown back (and often it can, with some of the newer drugs such as minoxidil, which we discuss in section Two) there are many other remedies. We will discuss them in sections Three and Four.

SECTION TWO

Growing It Back

CHAPTER 3

User Beware:
Some Common and
Not So Common Remedies

EVERYONE WITH A HAIR LOSS PROBLEM HAS HAD A FULL SHARE of advice from well-meaning friends, and from not-so-well-meaning charlatans. Most of it simply doesn't work. If you are suffering from abnormal hair loss, you probably need the advice and help of a doctor.

Your barber or hairdresser, or some other nonmedical hair expert, may be able to recognize problems arising from hair breakage, but they are not the people to treat hair loss or hair that fails to grow. They can often give you excellent suggestions for hair care, and may be the first to notice that your hair is thinning. (Section Six describes many of the recommendations they give their clients.) But beware of those who offer cures for pattern baldness. Some of these remedies, both new and old, can be worse than useless.

Vitamins

Vitamins that are sold as hair restorers will *not* arrest pattern baldness, nor will they cause regrowth. Good nutrition and vitamins can help your hair look better but that is all they can do. If a seriously inadequate nutritional intake or absorption problem has caused hair loss, hair will usually grow back when the problem or deficiency is corrected. Any one with a real nutritional problem should be evaluated by a physician.

Special Foods

Many health food stores sell a little booklet, now in its tenth printing, which suggests, among other things, that a low-salt diet, food rich in iodine such as kelp (dried seaweed), wheat germ, and a modest intake of animal protein will help prevent baldness. None of these suggestions have been confirmed by any documented studies. In fact, wheat germ may be beneficial for your general health, but is not so good for your hair! Norman Orentreich, M.D., Clinical Professor of Dermatology at the New York University School of Medicine, has had more experience treating, writing and talking about baldness than anyone else. He says that wheat germ is androgenic and that, potentially, it may aggravate hair loss rather than prevent it. Dr. Orentreich also cautions against excessive vitamin and mineral intake, because these can also cause or aggravate hair loss.

Scalp Massage

Proponents of scalp massage say that a major cause of pattern baldness is lack of blood circulating in the scalp region. They advise you to massage your head daily, using your fingers, a brush, or a vibrator-massager. Dermatologists, however, caution against vigorous massage. They state that it is useless, since there is sufficient blood in the scalp area (the chapters on transplant will clearly demonstrate this), and that massage can cause hair to break off at or near the roots. Many people feel that massage eliminates excessive oil, but frequent washing will accomplish this more effectively.

100 Strokes a Day

I grew up thinking that if I brushed my hair one hundred times a day I would have beautiful, shiny hair. Each year I would make a New Year's resolution to do it, but would then forget about it by mid-January. Before the introduction of modern shampoos, brushing helped remove soap residue, and thus made hair look shinier and brighter. But dermatologists and hair care specialists now tell us to forget the "100 strokes a day" adage. Indeed, excessive brushing can lead to breakage of the hair.

Heat Treatments

Heat treatments, either of the salon or home variety, can help hair that has been damaged by chemicals look and feel better. They will not, however, cause *new* hair to grow.

Slant Boards and Head Standing

Some self-appointed hair-growing experts recommend lying on a slant board—feet up, head down—or standing on the head. The theory is that it will increase the blood supply to the scalp, but no one has ever proved that slant boards or head standing stimulate hair growth.

Folk Remedies

An amazing number of so-called folk remedies and herbal cures are still sold by mail order and in health food stores. None of them will restore hair.

Oils, Lotions, and Creams

Even hair restorers that have been advertised for years are worthless, as anyone who has tried them can testify. They usually don't promise immediate results, so that by the time men (or women) who are suffering from pattern baldness realize the product doesn't work, they have spent hundreds of dollars and grown a bit balder. Many men are so eager to find a cure that they try one product after another.

Most of the companies who advertise their products are rather vague about the ingredients. Although the company will list some of them, they usually make claims that their product is the result of a "unique combination," and that it has shown "remarkable results in Europe." They never say who created the formula, or show any documented statistics regarding its efficacy.

Sometimes a special "total hair care salon" sells their own product, stating the treatment will cure baldness. The "before and after" pictures could fool just about anyone. In New York, one highly lucrative unisex hair care salon which offered various pricey treatments also sold their products for home use. Their spokeswoman, Ms. Galen (not her real name) was one of several hair care experts on a popular midday television show not so long ago, and I happened to be in the studio. Prior to the taping, two of Ms. Galen's clients showed me their "before" pictures. Indeed, their hair seemed to have grown thicker and fuller since the photographs were taken.

During the show I listened to Ms. Galen explain how her lotion, which consists of alcohol, witch hazel, and herbs, cleanses the hair and "unclogs the follicles, allowing the hair that is twisted inside the follicle to pop out." The studio audience, many of whom had little knowledge of hair growth, seemed impressed. But the physicians on the show, and a few call-in guests, quickly set everyone straight. They explained that scalp biopsies have never revealed curled or twisted hair in a follicle, and, as one call-in guest pointed out, if a hair was twisted inside a follicle it would create a visible lump.

Ms. Galen persisted in trying to prove that her methods work. "Look at my clients," she said, as the "before" pictures were flashed on the screen. The smiling, apparently full-haired guests nodded in agreement. "You see how their hair has grown," she stated. As the physician guest carefully examined each person's hair it became obvious to both the studio and home audiences that their *remaining* hair had been grown long and had been attractively styled to cover the bald and thinning areas. "Good grooming," he acceded to Ms. Galen. But hair growth, no. "Any good hair stylist could have achieved the same result for a lot less money."

Products and hyped-up sales pitches like the one Ms. Galen

gave abound all over the country. But now this is about to end.

The FDA Ban

A few years ago the Food and Drug Administration (FDA) invited companies to submit their products for evaluation. Few took up the offer, but the FDA remains convinced that all of these so-called over-the-counter products are worthless. Starting in 1986 the FDA will enforce a ban on all nonprescription baldness cures.

Does this mean there will be no more such products? Edward R. Nida of the FDA explained that the ban will pertain to any product that claims to *stop* hair loss, or to *restore* lost hair.

But what about products that simply describe themselves as conditioners and hair cleansers?

In several health food stores I visited I asked for something for baldness. In each store I was either handed a product or directed towards a selection of them. While in most instances the labels did *not* state that the product would grow hair, the intent was clear.

Will the FDA be able to ban these products? Probably not. Not if the manufacturer or distributor doesn't advertise or state on the label that the product will cause regrowth.

Manufacturers *will* have difficulty marketing products by mail, because the FDA will carefully monitor their advertising. Even if there are no promises or guarantees, if a photograph or illustration suggests the product is for hair regrowth, the FDA will clamp down on them.

Some products fall into the gray area between prescription and over-the-counter products. They may be sold in a clinic-like setting, overseen by a licensed physician, or given out by a physician's representative (such as a nurse, nursing assistant or technician). The FDA does not interfere if a physician distributes a product to individual patients whom he or she has evaluated and feels would benefit from a suggested product.

CHAPTER 4

Where's the Data?

TWO NONPRESCRIPTION PRODUCTS THAT HAVE GAINED A GREAT deal of attention in the press and elsewhere were developed by physicians, and have undergone some scientific scrutiny.

Although they seem to have been untouched by the FDA ban as yet, I was unimpressed with the statistics they presented, and when I asked some of the young men with whom I am acquainted to try the products, they did not find them helpful.

The Helsinki Discovery

In the 1970s, at the University of Helsinki Hospital in Helsinki, Finland, Ilona Schreck-Purola, M.D., a pathologist, and her associates were doing cancer research when they noticed that polysorbate, a common food additive that is approved by the FDA, caused hair to grow on bald white mice. In the way of so many accidental discoveries, the doctors in Helsinki realized they had stumbled onto a compound that might have potential for the treatment of baldness. Dr. Schreck-Purola and her associates decided to do further studies using the original compound which, in addition to polysorbate, included vitamins B_6 and niacin. The first studies conducted in Helsinki involved 40,000 mice, and the results were very encouraging. In a follow-up study of 320 people (47 women and 273 men) the formula stopped hair loss and/or caused hair regrowth in eighty percent of the subjects. Another study, done in France, resulted in similar findings.

How does this formula work? According to Dr. Schreck-Purola, polysorbate removes excessive cholesterol from the scalp cell membranes and aids in cell division, making hair regrowth possible. The concept, according to many physicians, is sound.

In the fall of 1984, Dr. Schreck-Purola visited Los Angeles, where she received a great deal of press. Some of the folks who tried it thought it was good. But now, a year later, when I contacted them they were disappointed and were seeking another method to reverse hair loss.

Making use of Dr. Schreck-Purola's findings, Hal Z. Lederman, president of Pantron 1, a California-based company, has formulated a treatment consisting of a shampoo, a conditioner, and vitamin pills, for distribution under the trade name of the Helsinki Formula.

A three-month supply of these products costs about $40. The conditioner lists its ingredients as purified water, polysorbate 60, biotin, niacin, methyl paraben and natural fragrances. The shampoo includes these ingredients plus wheat germ oil, vitamins, proteins and other ingredients for cleansing.

Testing the Helsinki Formula

Hal himself believes in the product, but to gain credibility he decided to conduct a study which would capture the attention of the media, even if it didn't convince the medical community. So in late 1984 he placed an ad in a newspaper in Bakersfield, California.

Wanted! 100 Bald or Balding Volunteers

for three-month test of the Helsinki Formula,

a new shampoo and hair conditioner.

The product was guaranteed as completely safe and each volunteer would receive a free three-month supply. Men and women aged twenty to sixty were accepted into the study regardless of the length of time or extent of their hair loss.

Hal told the volunteers that if they didn't see an improvement within the three-month test period they were not likely candidates for successful hair restoration. The volunteers were all photographed, and they agreed to complete a monthly questionnaire which would monitor their progress.

The folks at Pantron 1 admit that this was not a scientifically controlled experiment. Nonetheless, they were certainly pleased with the results of their three-month study.

Will the hair continue to grow? Stabilize? Or fall out? It is far too early to know.

Will the FDA put a stop to the Helsinki Formula? That depends on how the product is marketed. The labels on the plastic bottles of shampoo and conditioner merely call it the Helsinki Formula, listing ingredients and offering directions for use. There is no written implication that the product is to restore hair, but would you plunk down a lot of money for shampoo and conditioner unless you were hoping for some spectacular results—like new hair growth? Thus, it may be difficult for Pantron 1's marketing people to avoid the FDA's strict ban.

Helsinki on the Hudson

Hair Again, Ltd., which describes itself as a "full-service hair clinic...with a hair forever promise," is a multimodality facility just off Fifth Avenue in New York. They refer people to physicians for various procedures, which we will discuss in depth in later chapters. They also make hairpieces and sell shampoos, hair conditioners, treatments and vitamins.

The products are purchased via Canada, which receives them from Helsinki, by company founder Maurice Mann. The formula was initially obtained from Dr. Schreck-Purola, so it is probably the same or similar to the Helsinki Formula.

Has Hair Again conducted any studies to prove the efficacy

of these products? No. Nor does Mann promise that his product will grow hair. He admits that if they could do that for everyone, there would be no need for them to offer their other services.

These products appear to be safe enough, so that the man or woman suffering from pattern baldness who opts for one of the treatments we have described, or for others with similar approaches "has nothing to lose," as the FDA spokesman told me, "but his wallet."

Does It Work?

Is the Helsinki formula really effective? I have seen videotaped testimonials, and spoken to participants in the study, and I was impressed *until* one of my sons-in-law and some of his friends tried the formula. Unless a study is done under very carefully controlled conditions—hair counting, matched subjects (ideally, twins), and a complete examination which determines the cause of hair loss—no serious researcher can view the results as significant.

"Where's the data?", all the dermatologists I spoke with asked. "Can anyone replicate the study?"

The Helsinki Formula was not the only product about which I was to hear that refrain.

Biotin Products

Pilo-Genic dispenses a full line of hair products at its sixty-eight medically staffed treatment centers throughout the United States, United Kingdom, Canada, Australia, and the Caribbean. According to Anita Young, the president of Pilo-Genic Research Associates, Inc., "These products are formulated to control excessive hair fallout and stimulate regrowth of hair on men and women whose hair follicles may have begun the miniaturization process, but are still alive."

Ms. Young is the widow of the late Edward Settel, M.D., research consultant to Pilo-Genic and a Fellow of the American Academy of Family Physicians. He had spent much of his forty-five-year professional career in family and geriatric practice as well as pharmaceutical research.

We're talking big business here—and it is a company which was founded by a licensed, experienced physician and his wife. But ask most New York dermatologists about Pilo-Genic's biotin products for hair growth and they pause. Then they ask you to turn off your tape recorder and to not quote them by name. Why?

The doctors say they don't like the lack of scientific data, and that it's not common medical practice to refuse to tell the medical community exactly what is in a formula.

Secret Ingredient

It is his secret ingredient that makes his formula work, Dr. Settel said. He described it as a mini-emulsifier, part of a unique delivery system that allows a penetrating cream or lotion to painlessly and effectively carry the (hair-raising) formula directly into the cells of the hair follicles.

Sophisticated Approach

The company's approach is different from many others. This is no over-the-counter product or mail-order "snake oil." The FDA knows what is in the product, Dr. Settel said, and his products are only dispensed at treatment centers after each patient/client is carefully evaluated. Pilo-Genic sends many people along their way to dermatologists or to hairpiece makers, if their hair is too far gone.

Where's the Data?

Although the results of a study at fourteen of Pilo-Genic's own clinics conducted from 1974–1981 showed good results, "where's the data?" still rings in my ears. Dr. Settel had talked to some of the leading dermatologists, inviting them to conduct studies with his product. So far, there has been only one report from any independent study, and that was not impressive.

Will the FDA ban Pilo-Genic's Biotin products? Probably not. They don't advertise their product as a hair restorer; the products are not sold over-the-counter, and they make no promises. The FDA declares, "If a doctor or his representative wants to suggest, 'try this for a while and see if it helps your hair loss,' we don't interfere."

There are a number of prescription products about which other doctors—mostly dermatologists—have been saying, "Try this for a while, and see if it helps your hair loss."

Progesterone

In the late 1960s, Norman Orentreich, M.D., Professor of Dermatology at New York University Medical Center, pioneered the use of progesterone for arresting hair loss. Progesterone is the same hormone that, in women, prepares the uterus for the fertilized ovum, and maintains pregnancy. As Dr. Orentreich explains it, progesterone competes with 5 alpha reductase (the enzyme that transforms testosterone into it's derivative, DHT), thus reducing DHT. In a rather complicated fashion, this alters the hormonal balance in the follicles and allows the female hormones to offset some of the male hormones, thus reducing hair loss in pattern baldness.

But won't that cause a man to experience all sorts of secondary feminizing effects? To have a full head of hair sounds fine, but not if a man must lose his libido and potency. It might make him *look* like a great date, but he won't get too many return engagements.

Progesterone, indiscriminately administered, conceivably *could* have that effect, and also cause breast development. But that doesn't occur—certainly not under the supervision of a physician (usually a dermatologist) well versed and trained in the technique.

Lest you think you are about to get a shot of progesterone in the arm or derriere, let me assure you that is *not* the way the hormone is used for hair loss. Instead, it is applied topically (to the surface of the scalp) as a cream or ointment, and/or injected directly into the scalp. Dr. Orentreich, and most of the dermatologists with whom I have spoken, say that a male patient is given no more than a two-to-four percent progesterone tincture, and is advised to apply only 1 cc twice a day to the balding areas. Women are given smaller doses (no more than 2 percent progesterone) to avoid menstrual irregularities, which can occur if the drug is absorbed into the body. Women also receive far more diluted concentrations than men when they receive injections to the scalp.

Some dermatologists combine progesterone treatment with estradiol and other female hormones, and they report that this is quite effective in stopping hair loss. All these treatments require a great deal of patience on the part of both physician and patient. It can take a great deal of time to see results, if they come at all.

Some of the men and women I spoke with report they have been disappointed in hormonal treatment because it did not really prevent baldness. Many agree that treatment had postponed the inevitable, but not indefinitely.

So many dermatologists throughout the country prescribe hormonal treatments for hair loss that it has become "standard" practice. Yet their effectiveness has never been scientifically proven. Many doctors therefore say they will remain unconvinced until they see closely scrutinized, highly scientific studies.

Aldactone and Tagamet

Another drug which has demonstrated some effect in slowing down the balding process is a diuretic, spironolactone, more commonly known by its trade name, Aldactone. Some people with hypertension and hair loss have taken it and found that both of their problems were helped.

Cimetidine, an ulcer medication better known by its trade name, Tagamet, also seems to arrest hair loss. Both this drug and spironolactone, both of which are taken orally, must be prescribed by a physician. For some not fully understood reason, these drugs seem to have some ability to block 5 alpha reductase.

Are These Drugs Legal?

Since none of these treatments has been statistically proven to be effective, why doesn't the FDA challenge their use?

Because it is completely within the law. A doctor is allowed to give you a drug for conditions other than the ones for which it has been approved. More about that on page 66.

Progesterone is a chemical, and although a prescription is required, a physician can arrange for a local drug formulator to make it up for his or carefully selected patients. Or the physician can make it up in his office.

Does Progesterone Work?

Albert Lefkovits, M.D., an assistant clinical professor of dermatology at the Mount Sinai School of Medicine in New York, and an oft-quoted expert on skin and hair care, believes that progesterone has some beneficial effects. "But," he adds, "if something were really good, there wouldn't be any baldheaded dermatologists."

But now, one major drug company thinks they may be able to put hair on a lot of men, including those bald-headed dermatologists.

CHAPTER 5

Breakthrough: Minoxidil, the Big Surprise

BY NOW MOST PEOPLE HAVE HEARD OF MINOXIDIL. BUT ORIGI-
nally it came along as a big surprise to the medical profession.
Back in the 1970s doctors noticed something very unusual
in some patients who were taking a drug for severe hypertension. The drug, called minoxidil, is manufactured by Upjohn, one of the nation's biggest drug companies. The trade
name of the drug is Loniten, and it is effective in lowering
blood pressure by relaxing and enlarging certain small blood
vessels so blood flows through them more easily. However,
some people taking the drug reported side effects such as an
increase in heart rate, rapid weight gain, or lightheadedness.
And, eight out of ten patients noticed something very unusual. About three to six weeks after beginning treatment,
they discovered that their fine body hair was growing darker
and longer. Fine vellus hair seemed to be converted to darker,
coarser, terminal hair on the forehead and temples, between
eyebrows, on the upper part of cheeks, on the back, arms,
and legs.

And, on the scalp.

No wonder it became known as the "werewolf syndrome."
Naturally, a lot of people were disturbed by all this hair
cropping up where they least expected or wanted it. Some
people refused to take the drug. Doctors recommended con-

trolling the excessive growth with a hair remover or by shaving.

But some people were delighted. Men who had been bald or balding for years suddenly had hair. Postmenopausal women whose hair was thinning were pleased to find new hair growth.

How Does Minoxidil Work?

It didn't take long for the clever people at Upjohn to realize that if they could harness this strange side effect into a cure, or even a treatment, for baldness, they would have a real winner. No one was sure how (or even if) it really would work. One theory was that the drug dilated the blood vessels in the scalp, allowing a greater rate of flow. But this was not convincing, since other methods of increasing blood flow to the scalp have never been proven to increase hair growth. Other theories are that minoxidil prolongs the growing phase, and shortens the resting and shedding phase, in both those who are balding and those who have not yet started the process.

But in any case, Upjohn and a number of other serious researchers thought it was worth close scrutiny.

The earliest studies were done at the Wisconsin Regional Primate Research Center in Madison, where Dr. Hideo Uno is studying the stump-tailed macaque, a monkey which develops a monk-like bald spot when it is about four years old. Dr. Uno's theory is that follicles shrink every four or five years, then after a time come back to normal. In some instances they remain in their shrunken state.

Upjohn asked Dr. Uno to study the effect of the drug on his monkeys, and he and his researchers discovered that when they applied minoxidil to the stump-tailed macaques who had begun to bald, the balding process was reversed. Those monkeys who had not yet begun to bald responded to minoxidil by never beginning the process. "Minoxidil seems to act like a fertilizer for hair follicles," he says, although why or how is a mystery.

Early Tests on Human Scalps

Something that works for monkeys in a lab doesn't always work for humans. So, quietly, without any fanfare, Upjohn began doing some small clinical trials—applying the drug to people's bald heads. These early studies had to consider several questions.

- Could hair growth be stimulated where the topical minoxidil was applied?
- Could hair growth be limited only to the area where minoxidil was applied?
- Would it be effective for all causes of hair loss including alopecia areata and common baldness?
- Would hair growth be normal in appearance?
- Would the growth disappear when treatment stopped?
- Was it safe?

To test the drug, Upjohn asked dermatologists to try it with some of their patients. There was concern that the drug could be absorbed through the scalp, causing blood pressure to be lowered too much, and other adverse reactions, so early tests were done with fairly weak solutions. These results were not always impressive.

Nevertheless, many dermatologists became interested, and some of them tried it on their own heads and those of family members. Carefully, they monitored blood pressure, did electrocardiograms, chest X-rays, blood levels, urine analysis, and chemistries, to make sure that not too much of the drug was being absorbed into the system.

Articles began to appear in medical journals about stubborn cases of alopecia areata which responded to minoxidil, and when dermatologists met at medical meetings and conferences, they informally shared their experiences with each other.

Men who had long given up on mail-order lotions and potions were eager to try something "respectable." Anytime a local newspaper, radio or television show mentioned minoxidil, dermatologists would be besieged by phone calls from eager would-be patients. Some days, these doctors were so overwhelmed with inquiries that one said, "Established patients with serious skin problems simply couldn't get through on our phone." Others said that when they went to a party or on vacation they were afraid to reveal their medical specialty because minoxidil was all anyone wanted to discuss with them.

Full-Scale Study of Minoxidil

Doctors, as well as patients, awaited more news about the drug. After a number of preliminary studies, Upjohn decided in 1983 to run a full-scale, highly scientific, statistical study on the effectiveness of minoxidil in arresting hair loss and causing new growth. Twenty-two hundred patients at twenty-eight locations coast to coast would participate for one year. Upjohn would then analyze the data thoroughly. When the time came to announce the results, no one would be able to point at them and say, "Where's the data?" It would all be there.

Even before the one year study was completed, an official Upjohn spokeswoman for minoxidil, Jan AufderHeide, spent hours answering reporters' questions.

"Until the code is broken," she explained, "we really don't know the results."

"Code?" I asked.

"This is a double-blind study," AufderHeide explained. A double-blind study means that neither the physician nor the patient knows exactly what anyone is getting.

In the minoxidil study it worked this way. Upjohn sent the physician, usually a dermatologist in a large medical center, twelve bottles of solution for each patient in the study. Each bottle contained seventy cc and lasted one month. It came equipped with a one cc dropper, which the patient used to apply one cc of the solution to the balding area each morning and each evening.

There were three groups of patients in the study. One group received a placebo (a solution that looked the same as minoxidil, but was really an ineffective substance) for four months, and then switched to 3 percent minoxidil for the remaining eight months. The second group received 2 percent minoxidil for the entire year. The third group received 3 percent minoxidil for the entire year.

At the end of the year, each physician sent the data on the patients to Upjohn. The physicians, of course, didn't know which group each patient was in, because it was all coded.

Unofficial Results

But many of the physicians were also doing their own private studies, not using Upjohn's solutions but making their own from tablets or arranging with local pharmacies to make it. Although these physicians generally reported that one-third of the patients had "some" hair growth, many of these same patients said they didn't *look* like they had much more hair. Another third had vellus hair growth, and the other third had insignigicant or no growth. On the brighter side, physicians I spoke with reported that it was rare for patients to experience additional hair loss during the period they were using minoxidil.

Interest in the Business Community

Financial analysts heard that these studies were being conducted, and many enthusiastically recommended that their customers buy Upjohn stock. During the spring of 1984 when I first began researching this book, Upjohn stock was selling at 45, and by January, 1986, it had risen to 127. I felt foolish that I hadn't been smart enough to buy it when I first heard about it; but after initial hype by the media, reports of disappointing results began to hit the press and airwaves. "20/20" did a report on minoxidil, after which many viewers decided it wasn't for them. *Barron's* questioned long-term safety of the drug and pointed out that people will have to stay on it indefinitely to make any achieved results last.

Yet in December, 1985, Upjohn filed a new drug appli-

cation with the FDA for approval of their preparation, called
Regaine Topical Solution. If the FDA should decide to clear
it for marketing, as safe and effective for male pattern baldness, it will be available *only* by prescription. By 1987 or
1988 the FDA will deliver its verdict, and although Upjohn
is hopeful, many people I have spoken with are not.

Why Does Upjohn Want FDA Approval?

You may be wondering why, if minoxidil is already an FDA
approved drug, there is a need for a new drug application,
and FDA approval. To gain FDA approval, a drug is evaluated
and approved for safety *and* for effectiveness in treating that
which it is supposed to treat. But a physician can, at his or
her own discretion, prescribe a drug to be used for some
purpose other than that for which the drug company has
received FDA approval. As we have seen, physicians prescribe progesterone, Aldactone and Tagamet for hair loss.

However, let us imagine that a physician decided that
some drug usually used for epilepsy could be made into a
solution or cream and applied topically to remove your warts.
He could prescribe the drug for you, and if it didn't remove
your warts and caused serious skin irritation you could, if
you so wished, sue your physician for malpractice. But you
couldn't sue the drug company, because the FDA never approved its use as a wart remover and the company never
suggested you or your physician use the drug for that purpose.

In order to market Regaine Topical Solution as an antidote
for hair loss, Upjohn must prove its safety and efficacy for
that purpose and earn FDA approval, a process which may
take two years or more.

What About Now?

Until the drug is approved and readily available, either by
prescription or over-the-counter, can you get it? Probably,
since any dermatologist who is interested in prescribing it

for you can learn how to formulate it from a colleague who has been using it for a few years.

However, not every pharmacy can or will take the minoxidil tablets and make a nice clear lotion that you can put on your head. Today, most pharmacists only dispense pre-measured solutions, count pills and tablets, and verify physician directions and consumer understanding. Many also keep patient profiles to avoid drug interactions. But not too many pharmacists are still called upon to compound drugs with a mortar and pestle.

But some still do this regularly. Marcus Ross, R.Ph., and Joseph Policar, R.Ph., pharmacists and owners of Cambridge Chemists in New York, still remember how to make drugs the old fashioned way and they make up minoxidil for many patients whose dermatologists have prescribed it for them.

Mr. Ross, who has worked closely with dermatologists for close to a half century, says those who are under forty years old, and whose balding is of fairly recent vintage often show some results. Those people who are over forty or whose hair loss is of longer duration, show far less response. Some dermatologists report better results than others with their private patients, and Mr. Ross thinks that the reason has to do with the way the drug is compounded. It is important, he says, that the scalp absorb the drug efficiently and comfortably. There are many solvents that allow the drug to penetrate the first layer of skin, but cause great irritation. Others may cause toxicity. He and some of the doctors with whom he works have experimented with a variety of penetrating solvents.

No one wants to walk around with a lot of gooky stuff on their heads, so after the tablets are pulverized (many pharmacists now use a coffee grinder instead of the old mortar and pestle) and combined with alcohol, propylene glycol, or other substances, the solution is filtered and sometimes suctioned, which more effectively purifies it and prevents any powdery residue from remaining on the head.

Participants in the official Upjohn study received the minoxidil solutions free, but for others this material doesn't come cheap. The tablets themselves are expensive, and since the pharmacist isn't just counting them out, there is an additional charge for compounding the substance. Costs range anywhere from $85 to $300 a month for sufficient lotion of 3 percent concentration to apply to an "average" bald area. In the meantime, Upjohn, in a package insert, warns people against preparing their own minoxidil brew, "because systemic absorption of a topically applied drug may occur." A thorough reading of the insert could frighten away many would-be users. On October 15, 1985, the FDA took a firm stand on advising pharmacists not to prepare minoxidil as a topical solution.

Minoxidil Experts Speak Up

One of the physicians who conducted a study for Upjohn continues to spend a great deal of time answering questions from his colleagues and from reporters. He is dermatologist Joel J. Kassimir, M.D., of the Hair Clinic of the New York University Medical Center's renowned Skin and Cancer Unit, Department of Dermatology.

Dr. Kassimir seems fated to have become an expert on hair loss. His hair started to recede at seventeen, and his father had been bald since he was twenty-one. Baldness seemed to abound on both sides of his family, and some of his cousins also began the balding process at a young age.

While still in college, Dr. Kassimir read all the literature he could find on the topic, hoping that somewhere he would find a way to reverse the inevitable. "Maybe that's why I chose this area of specialty," he says with a boyish grin.

He feels that minoxidil is clearly the best thing that is available now. "It's not going to grow all sorts of hair on people's heads," he says, "and people in their thirties and forties shouldn't expect to grow full heads of hair.

"I have seen patients who grow nothing but a little peach fuzz, but to get a really good response, you have to have some hair with which to work. It doesn't seem to grow on a really bald head.

"One woman in our study was beginning to bald like a

man, and she grew it back! We thought, at first, that perhaps she had something other than pattern baldness, and we did several scalp biopsies on her. But in the histology reports all came back, 'pattern baldness.'"

Dr. Kassimir explained about the strict criteria for participation and follow-up in the official Upjohn study. There was no hanky-panky here. Baldness had to be measurable by a specific scale. A receding forehead wasn't sufficient: there had to be measurable hair loss at the crown. Caucasians, Hispanics and black men and women were included in the study but because blond hair loss doesn't photograph accurately, blondes were left out. Because the study is a blind one, Dr. Kassimir doesn't know whether those participants who continued to bald had received the placebo for a few months, or the 2 percent or 3 percent formula.

But he does know about his own head. He himself has been using minoxidil for a few years, and he hasn't lost any more hair. Of course, we must remember that unless Dr. Kassimir had a twin brother on whom the drug *wasn't* used, we will never be sure he would have balded *without* the drug.

Dr. Kassimir anticipates using the drug indefinitely, but with less frequency, or until something even better comes along. He already uses less of it than he did when he began treatment, and he feels, as do some of the other dermatologists who have talked with me about it, that after hair grows in patients will be able to remain on a modified "maintenance program."

Another much interviewed minoxidil expert is Michael Lorin Reed, M.D., clinical assistant professor of dermatology at New York University Medical Center. Dr. Reed was contacted by Upjohn in 1979 to work on some of their early studies to determine the safety and effectiveness of the drug. He used it on patients in his office, as well as on his own head. He says that he has seen some really fine results in people with thinning hair, but he thinks that it may be necessary to continue treatment for long periods of time—probably indefinitely. "It is still too soon to tell," he says, "but we do know that in those people who took the drug for their high blood pressure, the new hair growth it caused began to fall out within two to six months after treatment was ended."

Many internists I interviewed in early 1986 spoke cautiously, and some negatively, about using the drug for hair loss. Generally, their feeling was that the potential risks and cumulative risks of the long-term use of the drug outweighed the benefit of the unimpressive hair growth they had seen.

Melvin Kahn, M.D., a cardiologist who is an associate clinical professor of medicine at Mount Sinai School of Medicine said, "I wouldn't use it on my head (and I'm starting to bald), nor would I recommend it to a family member."

Lawrence R. Krakoff, Professor of Medicine at Mount Sinai School of Medicine and chief of the division of hypertension, has had a great deal of experience prescribing minoxidil internally for severe cases of hypertension. He too is worried about long term risks of using it topically for hair loss. He feels that a compound that is as active as minoxidil could present "as yet unknown risks," and he would advise people with hair loss not to use the drug for that purpose. He feels that men who do use it will be "condemned to long term use," because all evidence indicates that when the drug is stopped, any hair growth that has been achieved will be lost.

Ronald Savin, M.D., clinical professor of dermatology at Yale University Medical School in New Haven, was an official Upjohn investigator who used the drug on his private patients as well. He said that results were disappointing in those with shiny bald heads but that in those with some hair, results were noted, "even if it were just a little peach fuzz."

Elise Olsen, M.D., assistant professor of dermatology at Duke University, has published findings in which she notes that minoxidil stimulates hair growth response. However, Dr. Olsen and her coauthor, Madeline Weiner, R.N., point out that it all depends on how you define response.

Most men I meet define response as hair you can really see, and are disappointed with the minoxidil results. They describe that one-third response that most investigators report as far more impressive in statistics that on their heads. Theodore Tromovitch, M.D., clinical professor of dermatology at the University of California at San Francisco, says that one or two percent have phenomenal growth, but most patients will not have a significant cosmetic result. He emphasizes that the hair that grows in becomes fatter, thus looking like more hair even though there may not be any additional hairs.

Hillard Pearlstein, M.D., assistant clinical professor of dermatology at the Mount Sinai School of Medicine and Robert Auerbach, M.D., clinical associate professor of dermatology at New York University Medical Center share a busy dermatology office in New York. They have been treating hair loss problems for many years and offer many different treatments including transplant surgery (see chapter six). They have been using minoxidil with their private patients for a few years, and have seen some impressive results in women.

The opinions from those physicians who are official Upjohn investigators and those who are using minoxidil in their private offices range from disappointment to cautious optimism. Much of the initial enthusiasm I heard in 1984 was no longer present in 1986, although there was some agreement that minoxidil was effective in arresting hair loss. All of the experienced physicians were concerned that patients might somehow obtain the drug in excessively strong solutions which might grow hair, but could cause dangerous side effects.

By the time the Upjohn study had concluded, but before the results were announced, many dermatologists and general physicians began to prescribe minoxidil. Some brazenly ran ads in newspapers and magazines promising a proven treatment for baldness. Yet many physicians who were initially excited and enthusiastic about minoxidil were frankly disappointed.

"Yes, it grew hair," said one physician who asked not be named. "Yet most of my patients, after their initial excitement at seeing some hair growth, felt it was really unimpressive and that they still looked bald or balding."

Gone Today, Hair Tomorrow

Some patients were impressed.

Kevin's bright red hair was thinning, and his hairline was receding quickly. He didn't get into the official study because his crown was still intact, but Kevin was worried. He had inherited his maternal grandfather's red hair and freckles, and it was beginning to look like he was about to fall legacy to Grandpa's shiny bald head as well. His dermatologist in California, an Upjohn investigator, was also using the solution on his private patients. So Kevin got the full treatment.

He didn't tell anyone—not even his girlfriend—and she was the first to notice. "Kevin," she said, one night when she was ruffling her hands through his hair, "I think it's growing. Your hair, I mean."

If you ask Kevin what he thinks of minoxidil he'll tell you he thinks its the greatest thing to come along since the wheel.

Chuck is a New York actor who has appeared in many television commercials, soap operas and a few major films. He's the kind of actor they cast in the role of the guy who gets the girl. He's tall, dark, and handsome—with a nice full head of hair. At least, from the front he has a nice head of hair. But when the camera shoots from the back, that thinning crown becomes very apparent. So off he went to one of the Upjohn investigators who was using minoxidil on his private patients. Chuck got the full treatment—3 percent minoxidil solution—and within a few short months enough hair had regrown so that the camera no longer revealed a thinning spot. Chuck is ready to vote an Oscar, Tony and Emmy to his dermatologist. And he bought 100 shares of Upjohn stock with the check for his latest beer commercial.

Flo's hairstylist first noticed her thinning hair. It wasn't falling out at a greater rate than usual, but it just didn't seem to be growing back the way it used to do. Changing her hairstyle helped a bit, but the high forehead and thinning crown couldn't be fully camouflaged. So Flo went to see the dermatologist who had been so helpful to her son when he went through adolescent acne. The "family dermatologist" as she likes to call him, sent her off to one of the Upjohn investigators in a nearby midwestern city, and this dermatologist started her on minoxidil lotion. Flo says, "I would have been satisfied if the balding process had just stopped— but when some additional hair began to grow I was ecstatic."

But for every Kevin, Chuck, and Flo, I met scores of disappointed and disillusioned minoxidil users who had such poor results that they regretted the time and money spent, hoping for a miracle.

Some, like Greg, a young computer programmer, who after months and months of treatment at a cost of $1000 *still* hasn't regrown any hair, finally gave up. And Sam, a college student, spent still more, to no avail.

Other Products on the Horizon

Lederle, another major drug company, is also working on a drug to counteract baldness. It is called viprostol, and it is a synthetic prostaglandin, applied topically to bald areas of the head. Prostaglandin, a hormone-like unsaturated fatty acid, is produced naturally in the body. As a drug, it can work like a vasodilator and, like minoxidil, has important effects in lowering blood pressure. Lederle is still a long way from offering the drug to patients and from seeking FDA approval.

No Miracle Cures

Will anything turn out to be the miracle for which men have waited centuries? Will we ever be able to stand in the back of the auditorium of a dermatologists' convention and not see any bald heads? Probably not. For even if the FDA does approve of minoxidil it should be remembered: It only grows hair on some people, and you will have to use it forever.

However, for all the men who want to get back yesterday's hair, there is still hope.

Hair transplants, and variations of them, are more successful than ever. Cosmetic approaches are so comfortable and natural-looking that only your hair stylist can know for sure. Most important, cosmetic approaches give instant hair. In the next chapters we will tell you more about the newest developments in reversing hair loss.

Putting It Back: Surgically

CHAPTER 6

Moving It
from Here to There

IN AN ERA WHEN KIDNEY, CORNEA, LUNG, LIVER AND EVEN HEART transplants have become almost every day occurrences, some people still haven't even heard about hair transplants. Or if they have, they think it is something quite different than it is.

Unlike major organ transplants, hair transplants are not donations from someone else. Instead they consist, quite literally, of moving, or transplanting, hair from one area of a person's head to another.

Back in 1963 when my balding friend, thirty-two-year-old Stan, announced he was going to have a hair transplant, I thought he was crazy.

"Move hair from the back of his head to the front!" I exclaimed. "Won't he start to lose *that* hair too?"

I was unaware of the principles of hair transplanting, in which little plugs of skin, scalp and hair follicles are moved along with the hair. These hair-bearing grafts are removed from the fringe area, (the area that isn't genetically programmed to bald) and placed somewhere else on the head. The hair continues to grow in its new location just as it would have done if it had remained in its original site.

This growth doesn't happen immediately. Actually, the hair falls out before it begins to grow. So when I saw Stan two weeks following surgery I thought his hairline looked just like my little daughter's favorite doll—*after* she decided to take it in the bathtub.

Three months later, Stan's transplanted hair was growing nicely, but he still had that doll's hair look. A year later he looked great, and he felt so much better about himself that I humbly admitted I had been all wrong. I wouldn't have viewed his plan as not only frivolous and impractical, but bordering on lunacy, if I had been better informed to begin with.

Now a handsome fifty-five-year-old grandfather, Stan has

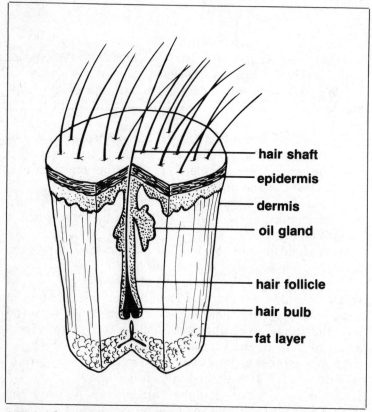

A Hair Plug Containing Follicle and Hair
The hair-bearing follicle is transplanted from the back or sides of the scalp to the bald area on the forehead or crown.

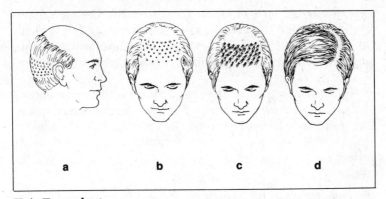

Hair Transplant
a) Donor plugs removed from fringe area, b) Plugs transplanted to top of head, c) Hair growth begins, d) Full growth of new hair merges with old

a hairline appropriate to his age. He is still pleased with his decision, and although he admits that in 1963 he had fantasies of looking like Robert Taylor, he soon came to terms with the fact that wasn't going to happen. He was content to look a lot better, and have enough hair so that no one, including his mirror, would label him bald. To keep up that look, Stan has had additional transplant sessions over the years.

Stan was among the early hair transplant patients. Now, almost thirty years after Dr. Orentreich of New York University Medical Center first began to use the technique, more than two million people (women, as well as men) have had the procedure. Dr. Orentreich reports it is the most commonly performed plastic surgery done today.

One of the reasons hair transplant is so popular is that it offers people the opportunity to have their own hair, which requires no special maintenance once healing occurs. Any barber or hairstylist can cut it. Providing there is sufficient donor hair to work with, hair transplant is suitable for anyone with permanent baldness caused by pattern baldness, scarring, accidents, surgery, radiation or congenital deformities.

Most hair transplants are done by dermatologists—probably because the procedure was first described by Dr.

Orentreich, a dermatologist. Traditionally, dermatologists have concerned themselves with various disorders of hair, but plastic surgeons, head and neck surgeons, and any other physician who has been trained in the procedure can perform it.

If the treatments described in section Two haven't worked for you, if you are unhappy with your permanent hair loss but want natural, permanent hair, you owe it to yourself to learn about and consider hair transplantation as a possible option.

Transplants Are Medical Procedures

Even before we further discuss transplants we need to remember—transplants are medical procedures. They should be performed only by a licensed physician who is trained in the procedure. Many hair clinics advertise that they are total clinics for hair care. They offer everything from simple styling to hair transplants. If they recommend a physician whom you call to schedule an appointment, this may be very satisfactory. However, if the clinic is unable to tell you who will do the procedure and doesn't provide you with any information on the credentials of the doctor—stay away. Transplants should not be done by a doctor who has read up a little on the procedure before moonlighting a few hours a week at one of these clinics. Chances are you won't even save any money by going to one of them, and you are at a double risk: medically and cosmetically.

Your own family physician or a friend who has had the procedure may be able to recommend a physician who does hair transplants. Some highly qualified physicians advertise, and you may see or hear one speak on a radio or television show. Sometimes doctors are mentioned in news reports or magazine articles. All the physicians quoted in this book are Board Eligible or Certified by the appropriate board of medical specialties, and have all graduated from accredited training programs. However, you should check the qualifications of any doctor who is going to do any sort of surgical procedure on you.

Is the doctor a graduate of an accredited medical school and has he/she completed a residency program in a teaching hospital? Is he/she a member of the staff of a good hospital? Is he/she Board Certified in a medical specialty? You can ask the doctor, but you can also get some of this information from your county medical society. Or your local librarian can help you find the reference books in which to check qualifications.

Everything You Ever Wanted to Ask About Hair Transplants Answered by Those Physicians Who Perform Them

Many people who are thinking about the possibility of a transplant have faulty notions both about the procedure itself, and the results. They may be fearful that it is very painful, or believe that it's no more uncomfortable than a teeth-cleaning session in the dentist's office. They may think it is either artificial looking, or an absolute panacea to their problems. They may have heard that they will have "instant" hair, or be fearful that transplanted hair won't grow.

To clear up the confusion, I have asked some of the physicians who perform transplants to share their experience and know-how. These dermatologists and plastic and facial surgeons include Doctors Robert Auerbach, Robert Berger, Richard Hamburg, Elliot Jacobs, Joel Kassimir, Donald Levine, Norman Orentreich, Hillard Pearlstein, Darrell S. Rigel, Ronald Savin, James Storer, D. Bluford Stough III, and Charles Vallis. Others have written for the general public and their material proved helpful. They are Doctors Herbert S. Feinberg, Richard W. Fleming, Toby G. Mayer, Walter P. Unger and Steven A. Victor.

The questions and answer section that follows is a synthesis. Doctors vary in their particular techniques, and all tailor their procedures to meet the individual needs of the patient.

What is a hair transplant?
It is a minor surgical procedure in which hair-bearing follicles, including skin, and scalp grafts are moved from one

area of the head to another area. These grafts, usually small four millimeter (⁵⁄₃₂ inch diameter) plugs, are taken from the back of the head in the area that is not genetically programmed for baldness. They are moved to areas that are balding or completely devoid of hair. Each plug yields approximately ten hairs.

How is the procedure performed?
The donor area at the back of the scalp, from where the hair-bearing follicles will be taken, is injected with a local anesthetic similar to that used by a dentist. The donor-site hair is then clipped short so that the doctor can see its angle and direction. Using an electric or hand-powered circular punch instrument that looks like a cookie cutter, the doctor gently removes the small scalp grafts containing the hair and follicles. The graft is then trimmed of excess fat and placed in a sterile saline solution.

Meantime, the recipient area (the bald or balding areas into which the hair will be grafted) has also been injected with a local anesthetic. With the circular punch, the physician removes small cylinders in the designated bald area. The recipient spaces are slightly smaller than the donor plugs, to ensure a close fit. This also minimizes scarring.

When the process is completed the physician places a nonadhering pressure dressing on the surgical area, which is covered by a turban-like bandage. These dressings are removed the following day.

I have heard these grafts called by various names: plugs, microplugs, strips. What are the differences?
Essentially they are all grafts. The word *plugs* refers to the usual three to five millimeter graft which is punched out of one area of the scalp and transplanted into another.

Charles Vallis, M.D., renowned plastic surgeon, who is on the faculty at both Harvard Medical School and Tufts Medical School, prefers four-and-a-half millimeter plugs to the usual four millimeter ones that most transplant surgeons use, because they can yield fifteen to twenty hairs. He also likes to cut the four millimeter plugs into small sections, each of which yield a few hairs per section. These *microplugs* are then placed between the larger plugs in the hairline, to achieve a more natural hairline.

Strips are just what they sound like. A strip of scalp with the hair-bearing follicles is removed from the back of the head and placed on the forehead to create a new hairline. The strips are usually very narrow, measuring less than a quarter-inch wide, and up to eight inches long. Dr. Vallis, a champion of strips, explains that they enhance the hairline when placed in front of the smaller plugs.

Some doctors are not as enthused: they think that strips are not as natural looking as the smaller plugs and they don't use them.

Where is a hair transplant procedure performed?
It is done in a doctor's office. There is no hospitalization involved at all.

Is this a painful procedure?
Most patients compare it to a session in the dentist chair. As you know, some people find a dental session more uncomfortable than others do. And some dentists cause less hurt than others.

So it is with hair transplants. The use of the local anesthetic deadens the area sufficiently that there is very little pain. Yet some people say there is considerable discomfort. Others are relaxed and comfortable and even doze off during the procedure.

Is it possible to have something stronger than the local injection of anesthesia?
Many physicians also offer patients a mild sedative, such as Valium, and/or a powerful painkiller like Demerol, administered orally or intravenously. A few physicians use nitrous oxide (laughing gas) during the procedure.

Those physicians who are skilled and experienced at the procedure find that patients have relatively little pain.

Am I good candidate for this procedure?
If your hair loss is due to pattern baldness, or is permanent
as a result of burns, accidents, surgery and radiation, or certain diseases or infections, you may be an excellent candidate. However, there must be sufficient hair to spare from an
area of the scalp that is not genetically programmed for baldness. In men, it has to be taken from the horseshoe rim at
the back of the head. Women can sometimes safely spare
some of the hair that is higher up.

Even if the ratio of baldness to available grafts is such that
coverage would be insufficient, that does not preclude transplant surgery. The transplant can be done in conjunction with
scalp reduction, which is discussed on pages 94–96.

Your general health must also be considered. If you suffer
from diabetes or any severe heart disease you may not be a
good candidate for this surgery. The transplant surgeon will
probably want to discuss any medical problems with your
family doctor or internist prior to making a decision.

Is it possible to be too young?
Even young children can have transplant surgery to correct
baldness caused by congenital conditions, surgery, accidents
and other trauma.

If you are in your early twenties and your hair loss consists
only of a receding forehead, it might be wise to wait until
the loss has extended; otherwise your new transplanted hairline may look unrealistically low when you get older.

However, baldness does not have to be fully stabilized
before a transplant is done, as long as you realize that you
may need more transplants in the future.

Is it possible to be too old?
Not if you have enough hair to spare, and your expectations
are realistic. If your doctor feels that your health is satisfactory, you can certainly be considered as a candidate for hair
transplant. However, a man must realize that if he doesn't
have a lot of hair to transplant, or if it is very thin, it will
remain sparse. But it can be more evenly distributed, and if
you style it properly it will look fine.

I don't have enough hair—but my sister has kindly volunteered to donate some of hers. Will that work?
Unfortunately it won't. Hair transplants are actually a form of skin transplant and the risk of rejection is as high as it would be for any other organ. When transplants are medically necessary, recipients are given drugs to suppress their immune system. This helps to avoid rejection, but such drugs carry a certain amount of risk, and are not appropriate for hair transplant surgery.

An identical twin would probably make a fine donor and you are unlikely to reject the transplant. But if your hair loss is due to pattern baldness, rather than to an accident or disease, your twin probably has no more hair to spare than you do!

Would it be possible to transplant hair from another part of the body, such as the chest?
It is possible, but highly impractical. And it would be unnatural in appearance. The hair growth would be sparse, kinky and very short.

Will the texture of my hair be suitable?
Thick or curly hair often looks best because it seems to take up a lot of space. Thin, light colored, sparse hair may not seem to cover your head as effectively, but it is acceptable to use it.

I scar easily—will that be a problem?
It might be, although some people who scar elsewhere on the body don't seem to have a problem with transplants. If you have had a history of scarring, your doctor will want to do one test graft to see how you respond.

Does a hair transplant always take?
When it is done by an experienced, well-trained physician, the success rate is excellent. Some hairs and an occasional plug may be lost in the transplant process, but it is the rare exception when most of a transplant doesn't take.

How can I be sure I have enough blood supply to nourish the grafts?
You do. Contrary to popular belief, even the bald scalp has an excellent blood supply.

How long will the hair last?
Indefinitely. The hair follicles are taken from the part of the scalp that never balds, and these transplanted follicles behave exactly as they would if they had remained in their original site. The transplanted follicles don't "know" they have been moved to an area of the scalp that usually balds. Instead they "think" they are still back where they started life.

Will the area from which the hair is taken look straggly?
No, because the donor grafts are spaced far enough apart so that the remaining hair grows over them. When done properly, it is almost impossible to see where the hair was removed.

Will new follicles, and thus new hair, regenerate in the donor area?
No. There are only a finite number of hair follicles, and if you take them from one area, they are gone. Thus, if thirty follicles are removed from the donor site, there will always be thirty less follicles there.

Will I eventually run out of hair to be transplanted?
That is a possibility. Sometimes when a patient begins the transplant process he has plenty of hair to spare to cover the bald areas. But over the years he may bald at a greater rate than even his physician anticipated, and if he still wants a fair amount of hair, there may just not be enough. This is an important consideration, and some men who have been through several transplants decide eventually that they still don't have enough hair and may combine transplant with a cosmetic approach or switch over to the cosmetic approach completely.

Where, exactly, will the transplanted hair be placed?
It will depend upon whether you have enough donor hair available to cover all your bald or sparse areas. If not, your doctor will consider your personal preferences. Some people are more concerned about the hairline, others about the crown.

Usually the first grafts are placed in the hairline area, in order to establish the new hairline. Later grafts are placed behind the hairline.

A man's hairline recedes somewhat as he ages. So a hairline should never be placed so low that it will look unnatural as you age. Remember that the transplanted hair will be permanent, and a hairline that is natural looking at twenty-five, will no longer be so in a man of fifty or sixty. Thus, it is usually necessary to compromise on where the hairline should be placed, especially if you are fairly young when the procedure is initially done.

Will a hair transplant look natural?
If you opt for a casual hairline, it can look fairly natural and will not be noticeable. Hair that is transplanted to the crown looks more natural (especially if it has a little length or is curly) than the hair that is transplanted to the forehead. A slicked back hair style may reveal the plugs if they are on the forehead, and if you are expecting to have a full head of hair you will be disappointed. A transplant can give you a good frame, and the look of no baldness, but it won't make you look like Robert Redford—or even Ronald Reagan (who really does have all his own hair).

What are the first steps to take if I am considering a hair transplant?
You should first meet with a doctor to discuss feasibility. Together, you will review the cosmetic approaches and results you both wish to achieve.

Once the date for the first session is set, how will I need to prepare?
Prior to the procedure, you may be told to shampoo your

hair thoroughly, in order to diminish oiliness and reduce the possibility of infection. Because aspirin can interfere with blood clotting, you will be told to avoid it for a week before surgery. You also should not have alcohol on the day of the surgery. Most doctors will suggest you eat something, but no more than a light meal prior to the surgery.

Be sure to wear a front-buttoned shirt on the day of your operation. You should not put anything over your head for several days after surgery to avoid damage to the grafts.

Should I have a haircut before the session?
No. You will want all your available hair to cover the donor and recipient areas until healing has taken place.

Will I have stitches?
There are two schools of thought and practice on this. Some physicians feel stitches control postoperative bleeding, hasten healing and lessen scar tissue. Other physicians feel stitches are superfluous, that healing is perfectly satisfactory without them. Stitches are occasionally placed in the recipient area.

Will there be much bleeding?
The scalp has many blood vessels, thus there is bleeding during the procedure. However, there will be little or no bleeding postoperatively.

Will I be sitting or lying down during the procedure?
Some doctors prefer to have patients sitting, barber-chair style, permitting better access to the head. Others prefer to have their patients lie down. Some arrange for the patient to lie down for most of the procedure, then sit for part of it.

How long will the procedure take?
Depending on the number of grafts and the rate at which your doctor proceeds, it can take from one to two-and-a-half hours. If the doctor works with nurses or trained technicians who help to prepare the plugs, this can speed up the procedure. However, since precise placement and correct an-

gling of the plugs is of paramount importance in achieving a natural look, only a highly trained person should do the actual placement of the grafts in your scalp.

How many transplants in all can a person have?

That, of course, depends on the amount of hair you have to spare. You may need six hundred to eight hundred plugs to cover one third to one half of your head. But for many people, one hundred to one hundred fifty plugs can effectively fill the crown and give a satisfactory hairline.

Will I have all the transplants done in one session?

Usually not, unless you are only covering a very small area that requires only about twenty or thirty grafts in all. Anywhere up to one hundred plugs can be transplanted at one session, but most physicians say that eighty is the maximum that should be done at one time.

Many physicians feel that healing is better if some space is left between each graft, so they prefer to transplant in two or more sessions—doing no more than fifty plugs at one time. This schedule allows one group of grafts to heal before the next group is transplanted.

How often can transplant procedures be done?

Many physicians prefer to wait three to four months between procedures if the grafts are to be placed in the same general area. This allows time for circulation in the area to return to normal. If the area to be transplanted is on a different part of the scalp, the intervals between procedures can be much shorter.

Will I have hair immediately?

Yes, and no. You will have hair immediately, but the transplant process is a shock to the hair follicles, forcing growing hairs into the resting phase. This results in shedding a few weeks after the transplant surgery. A small amount of hairs may be permanently lost, but most of the shed hair will begin to grow back at the usual rate of about one half inch a month.

One of the Upjohn minoxidil investigators, Darrell S. Rigel, M.D., Clinical Instructor, Department of Dermatology at New York University Medical Center, did an interesting study. Starting one week after transplant and continuing for twelve weeks, patients applied minoxidil twice daily to their grafts. He noted that almost half of the hair continued to grow, rather than shedding as described above. Very little hair (far less than usual) was permanently lost, leading Dr. Rigel to conclude, "Minoxidil may be additive in its effect to hair transplant." Both Drs. Rigel and Kassimir will be conducting a "double blind" study for Upjohn to see if this observation is accurate.

Dr. Ronald Savin of Yale has made the same observation, and predicts that the combination of transplant and minoxidil may be the wave of the future, leading to even better results than have previously been achieved.

Will there be any scabs or crusts on the grafts?

Yes, scabs or crusts are formed over both the donor and recipient graft sites, forming a natural protective covering. They remain from one to three weeks after transplant surgery, and then will be shed along with the transplanted hairs. At that time, the scalp is usually well healed. Scabs can be minimized by good surgical technique, by cleansing the scalp with peroxide the day after surgery, and by early but careful shampooing.

After surgery will I be able to return to my usual activities?

Some people have the surgery in late afternoon, go home, eat dinner with their family, have a good night's rest, and return to their office the next morning.

Your doctor will want you to avoid major physical activities for the few days following surgery, so if your job requires a great deal of strenuous activity you may need to take some time off from work. Although activities and exercise are limited for the next week or ten days, transplant surgery is in no way incapacitating.

Will there be any pain after the procedure?

Like the procedure itself, this is an individual matter. Your doctor will suggest a mild, non-aspirin analgesic following surgery. Few people need anything stronger than that.

Some people say they have a dull headache for a few weeks following the surgery, which is easily relieved by mild analgesics. A numbness in both the recipient and donor graft areas may persist for some time, but it will eventually go away.

Will there be some special instructions on the care of my head following surgery?
The bandages are removed the day after surgery either by you or the doctor, at which time some physicians like to clean the surgical site. If by any chance a plug needs to be reoriented it can be done at this time. If you have nondissolving stitches, they will be removed one to ten days after the surgery.

You may be given an antibiotic ointment to put on the grafts, to keep them soft and prevent infection. You will be told not to disturb them or run a comb or brush over them for two weeks.

The scalp can be gently shampooed with a mild shampoo sometime between the third and tenth days. You may also be able to go swimming at that time.

Excessive sun should be avoided because the new skin, which has been on the back of the head, has not previously been exposed. Gradual tanning is permissible.

Do infections sometimes occur?
Very seldom. If an infection should occur, it is easily treated with antibiotics.

Do any of the grafts ever fall out?
Occasionally. Some physicians may give you instructions on saving them.

Will there be any bleeding after the surgery?
If there is any bleeding it can be easily controlled by the application of firm, moderate pressure directly on the site for fifteen minutes, using gauze or a clean handkerchief.

Avoiding aspirin and alcohol for the first few days after surgery will help to prevent bleeding.

Am I likely to have any swelling?
Your physician will probably suggest you sleep with an extra pillow to avoid swelling. One to four days after the procedure, some painless swelling may develop at the recipient area, on the forehead, over the bridge of the nose or in the eyelids. Cool-water compresses, remaining erect as much as possible, and sleeping with extra pillows will relieve the swelling, which in any case usually disappears in two to three days.

Will I take any medication other than non-aspirin analgesics following the procedure?
Some physicians prescribe antibiotics to prevent infections, or cortisone to avoid swelling.

Is there some way to camouflage the "unfinished" look until hair begins to grow in?
Yes, indeed. You can wear a hat or a hairpiece.

Will there be visible scars after surgery?
There is some scarring, in both the donor and recipient areas. These scars tend to improve with time, and are covered by the hair. However, people whose hair is very light colored and thinning may find that camouflage is harder to achieve.

Sometimes, the transplanted grafts are slightly elevated, giving a cobblestone effect. Meticulous surgical technique minimizes this problem, but if it occurs, cauterization will flatten the elevation.

Will the skin that is grafted along with the hair match the skin on my forehead?
It may look different at first. Since your forehead has been exposed to sun and wind, and the skin in the back has been protected by your hair, there may be a slight difference in color. Gradually, they will blend, and a few summers of slow

sun tanning will provide an even better match. The hair will cover the area, so it is unlikely to be noticeable.

Are complications possible?
No one can guarantee there will be none, but the complication rate in hair transplants is very low when performed by a well-trained, experienced physician.

How much will it cost?
There is a range in costs for transplant surgery. Most doctors charge per plug, ranging from $20–$35. Surprisingly, some of the most experienced and best regarded doctors in the field charge no more (and maybe even less) than some of the ones who advertise heavily and are not as experienced.

At $25 a plug, this is still a fairly expensive procedure. A fairly balding person may require 500 plugs, at a total cost of $12,500.

Will my health insurance plan pay for it?
Rarely, unless the procedure is done to correct an accident or illness. When performed strictly for cosmetic purposes, hair transplant (and the other procedures we will discuss in this and the next chapter), like most cosmetic plastic surgery, is seldom reimbursable under medical plans.

Will "Uncle Sam" agree that it is tax deductible?
Hair transplants (including the procedures we will discuss in this and the next chapter) have been, in most instances, an acceptable medical tax deduction.

Suppose I'm miserable with the results, am I stuck with it?
Not entirely. Electrolysis can remove the hair, but it is a very uncomfortable, painstaking, and not always successful procedure.

This is why it is important to give it a great deal of thought. Observe and speak with people who have had the procedure, and thoroughly "check out" the doctor's credentials and reputation. Pictures can be deceiving, so ask any doctor with whom you consult if you can personally see some of his/her patients.

Hair transplants are not for everyone. A person must be highly motivated to have the surgery, and should not do it just because his wife or someone he cares about thinks it's a good idea. He himself must feel strongly that he wants hair—his own permanent hair—and is willing to spend the time and money required to achieve it.

Hair transplant is seldom a one-time or even two-time procedure. In all likelihood, you will want or need additional procedures over a period of time, as further balding takes place.

Scalp Reduction

You now know just about everything you need to know about the punch-plug graft transplant technique. But you may have one more important question: "Is there anything that can be done for someone who has too *much* scalp, as well as too *little* hair?"

To rephrase it, you may have hair to spare, but not enough to cover that bald area. But, now at last, there's hope even for people who have that problem.

Scalp reduction, or alopecia reduction as it is often called, is sometimes described as the most significant development in the surgical treatment of baldness since the punch graft transplant. In this procedure, portions of the bald scalp are removed, and the elasticity of the skin allows the remaining scalp to be pulled together and surgically stitched.

This makes the bald area smaller. It also means that in the transplant surgery that usually follows scalp reduction, fewer grafts are needed. Therefore, men with large areas of baldness may, with reduction, now have sufficient donor hair to provide coverage. The procedure is especially valuable for younger patients whose baldness is likely to develop further, since more of the donor area can be saved for future use.

Scalp reduction is a relatively painless office procedure, although some physicians prefer to do it in the hospital. The

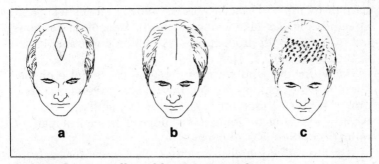

Scalp Reduction Followed by Hair Transplant
a) Excision of scalp in a man with large area of baldness, b) Skin pulled together and sutured, reducing area of baldness, c) Plugs transplanted on reduced bald crown

surgeon makes two longitudinal cuts in the scalp, removes and discards the skin in the mid-section, and sews the ends together. The amount of skin excised is dependent on the looseness of the skin, but a width of up to two inches can be done at one time. If there is considerable baldness, the process is repeated at six to ten week intervals to achieve a satisfactory result. Although scalp reduction will reduce the area of baldness considerably, it cannot completely eliminate it. For full coverage, some form of transplant must follow.

The amount of anesthesia needed during reduction surgery varies according to the doctor's assessment of the individual patient. Local anesthesia, sometimes combined with intravenous Valium or Demerol, and occasionally nitrous oxide, provides sufficient blocking of pain.

Following the surgery, antibiotic ointment is applied and the scalp is bandaged. The patient removes the bandage the following day, and continues to apply an antibiotic ointment to the suture area for two weeks. Oral antibiotics are often given to patients. The stitches are removed by the physician a week to two weeks following the surgery.

There may be some swelling within a few days after the procedure, but any pain or discomfort will respond to analgesics. A scar will remain where the scalp has been sutured together, but it will be covered by either the surrounding hair, or by the hair-bearing grafts. Some surgeons wait until after healing has taken place to begin transplant sessions, but others do both procedures—reduction and transplant—at the same time.

Some doctors who perform transplants are not enthused about scalp reduction, saying that it is an overused procedure. They argue that if the skin isn't sufficiently loose, there is only a saving of about fifty plugs. For such a patient, reduction offers few advantages.

Is scalp reduction cost effective? Costs vary for scalp reduction, but are generally in the area of $1,500. If you save only sixty plugs at $25 each, there is no momentary advantage. But reduction can add considerably to the cosmetic result.

Scalp Stretching

Donald Levine, M.D., a facial plastic surgeon, is associated with Manhattan Transplant, a New York medical office that specializes in hair transplant. Dr. Levine and his staff perform many hair transplant procedures and they are very excited about their new scalp-stretching method for those patients whose scalps lack elasticity, and so are not ideal candidates for reduction prior to transplant.

To achieve this scalp stretching, Dr. Levine makes a small incision in the scalp, then inserts two silicone inflatable bags under the scalp. Over a period of four to eight weeks, he gradually fills the balloon-like bags with sterile saline water. As the skin stretches it becomes more elastic. When the skin has stretched sufficiently, the bald area can be reduced, and transplant can follow.

At the International Congress for Hair Replacement Surgery, held in New York in the spring of 1984, Richard Anderson, M.D., of the Department of Plastic Surgery of the University of Michigan, discussed and demonstrated the scalp-stretching work he and Louis Argenta, M.D., have been doing. They find the scalp-stretching method excellent in children who have suffered permanent alopecia in one particular area. All or some of the bald area can be excised. Then, grafts can be used to fill in the remaining baldness.

The logic behind the concept is very sound. We know that during pregnancy a woman's skin can stretch tremendously. After she gives birth, the skin is slack and appears to have great elasticity.

There is one catch in this method for correcting pattern baldness. The balloons on either side of the head create two unsightly protrusions. If a person has a special occasion scheduled, the water can be drained out and replaced afterward, although some surgeons such as Elliot Jacobs, M.D., Manhattan plastic and reconstructive surgeon, say, "You lose ground that way."

"I was called a 'fathead,'" one man said, "but only temporarily." As soon as reduction surgery was performed, I looked perfectly normal. But with more hair than before."

This is an expensive procedure: the scalp-stretching methods plus the reduction can cost up to $5,000 or $6,000. The punch plug grafts that follow bring the cost up still more.

Scalp Flaps

Another method of transplanting hair actually gives instant hair. More difficult to perform, successful only in the hands of an experienced surgeon, this procedure is described as flap grafts.

The transposition flap, or scalp-rotation surgery for baldness, involves the cutting out of a large patch (1½–2 inches wide) of hair-bearing scalp, along with its own blood supply, and sewing it to the bald area of the scalp.

D. Bluford Stough III, M.D., Hot Springs, Arkansas, dermatologist, the former president of the American Association of Cosmetic Surgeons, believes that hair-bearing flaps are an extremely important advance in hair replacement surgery. "Patients with finely textured, sparse hair and those with limited hair who desire dense frontal coverage in the shortest period of time are excellent candidates for a flap procedure," he says.

In most instances the transplanted area is not removed

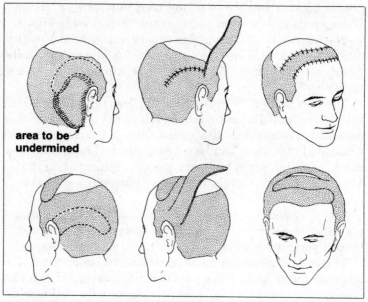

Transplant of Flaps of Hair-Bearing Scalp
In this sequence of pictures, you can see how flaps of hair-bearing scalp are taken from one part of the scalp and moved to another part. After the flaps are removed, the donor areas are pulled together and sewn, and the transplanted flaps are sewn to the bald area.

from the scalp, but is simply pivoted to another area. However, it is also possible to transplant a strip that has been completely detached from the scalp. The latter is called a free scalp flap. While it is more versatile than a rotated flap, it is essentially a graft, and this can more readily be lost, resulting in permanent loss of hair. Many experienced plastic surgeons only use the free flaps to correct serious cosmetic defects.

The rotating scalp flap procedure, when done properly, can achieve a great deal. Because the strip of hair-bearing scalp retains its own blood supply, it usually takes very well. Naturally, the distance that these flaps can move is limited because they must remain partially attached to their original site. For this reason, scalp reduction is often performed prior to flap transplants.

Only a handful of surgeons perform the hair flap procedure on a regular basis. If the procedure should fail it would leave the patient with less hair than he had before.

Advocates of flaps say that their great advantage is instant hair. This procedure seldom shocks the hair into the resting and shedding phase. And because there is a normal distribution, density and texture of hair, it can look even more natural than plugs.

There are several kinds of flaps:

Temporoparietal, or two short flaps, are patches extending back from above each ear. They are placed so as to meet each other in the front, forming a hairline. This may be done in one or two stages, and is usually performed in the office under local anesthesia.

Preauricular flaps are shorter flaps taken from in front of the ear and moved about two-thirds of the way toward the front of the scalp. This procedure is usually done in one stage, and is also performed in the office under local anesthesia.

The temporoparietal and preauricular flaps are sometimes done in conjunction with each other.

Juri flaps, named after the surgeon who introduced them, involves multi-stage, more extensive procedures than the other flaps. They require some hospitalization and general anesthesia. Many experienced plastic surgeons will not attempt the Juri flap, and some, like Dr. Vallis, describe it as a major operation and strongly advise patients to avoid it.

Those surgeons who perform flaps feel that the first two procedures, in particular, are highly reliable. But there is one major disadvantage. The hair doesn't always "go" in the right direction, and while this may be of no consequence on the crown, it can look unnatural at the hairline. Proponents of flaps say the misdirection of hair can easily be overcome with good styling, including permanent waving.

Flap surgery, as you have probably concluded, is an interesting and effective way of gaining instant hair. A more

extensive procedure than punch plug or strip graft transplantation, it sometimes results in some scarring. That is
because after the flap is moved, the remaining ends of the
skin are sutured together. However, hair will usually cover
it.

There is one major difference between grafts and flaps.
Grafts are a segment of tissue transposed from one area of
the body to another. They are completely removed in the
process and depend on the blood supply of the new, recipient
site. A flap is moved with all or most of its own blood supply
and, as usually performed, remains attached at one point to
its original site.

The risk of permanent loss of hair is greater in a flap than
with plugs. If one or two plugs don't take, you still have the
others. If, unexpectedly, a flap doesn't take, you have lost a
great deal of hair.

The cost of flaps is higher and, depending on the number
of procedures involved, can range from $1,500 to $15,000.

Making the Decision

How does a surgeon who performs all the procedures decide
which one is right for each patient? Some physicians say that
if a man has a large area of baldness and wants the frontal
hairline restored he should use hair flaps rather than grafts.
If there is a small area, or simply a part of the hairline that
needs filling in, then they recommend strips or plugs.

Dr. Joel Kassimir and many other surgically trained dermatologists feel that plugs continue to be the most effective
surgical method for hair replacement. "If you are truly an
artist," says Dr. Kassimir, "they take time to do well."

However, you may have to make the decision yourself.
Not all medical hair specialists perform all procedures. If
you go to a doctor or medical center which only offers one
type of procedure, a full range of options may not be available
to you.

Punch plug transplants and hair flaps are not for everyone.
If you have too little hair, or hair that is thin and light in

color, these methods may not be viable. Or, if you are determined to have a full head of hair, they will not give you what you want. But you can still have hair—and it can be firmly attached to your head. Some interesting new techniques combine surgical procedures with hair pieces, and in the next chapter we will describe them.

CHAPTER 7

Surgeons and Stylists: An Interesting Collaboration

THE QUEST FOR A FULL HEAD OF HAIR—ONE THAT LOOKS AND feels natural—is eternal. It was inevitable that the medical profession and cosmetic industry would collaborate to find a solution.

Some of the results of this collaboration have been acceptable—such as the cosmetic suture retainer process and tunnel grafts, which we will discuss in detail in this chapter.

But one such approach to instant hair was far less than unacceptable. It was disastrous, and some of the victims of the fiber implants, so popular in the 1970s, are still suffering the results of that procedure. Although the FDA has banned the procedure, and almost all of the states have passed laws against it, it is possible that some unwary customers are still being talked into the process by unscrupulous clinic proprietors.

Synthetic Fiber Hair Implants—a Warning

Although most physicians were skeptical, and some were immediately aghast, it sounded like a good idea—at first.

Thousands of synthetic strands, dyed to match a person's own hair, were implanted directly into bald areas of the head. In these fiber implant clinics, (occasionally supervised by a doctor), a technician used either a metal hand instrument or an air-driven gun to sew or insert the fibers into the scalp.

The process itself was painful because of the prolonged and repeated injections of local anesthetic, and it was often accompanied by considerable bleeding.

People tolerated the pain because they were so eager to have all that wonderful, instant hair. But later, their real trouble started. Within two or three weeks, the fibers began to break or fall out. Those which remained frequently caused intractable pain, facial swelling, infection, scarring, and loss of the person's own remaining hair. As fiber implant clinics proliferated, articles began to appear in medical journals about patients whose complications were so serious as to require skin grafts.

Dr. Wilma Bergfeld reported on the economic and psychological effects among forty-one Ohio patients who required treatment for medical complications of the fiber implants. "Many patients had self-image problems and long-standing psychological trauma following the procedure." The costs of the process had averaged more than $2,000 each, the patients lost time from work, and incurred huge expenses for continued medical treatment.

The attorney generals of many states sought and received injunctions against the proprietors of these clinics but most of the victims of fiber implantation never received any refunds. The FDA and the Federal Trade Commission received so many complaints that, in March 1979, the FDA issued a public warning about the implants. In June of 1983 the implants were officially banned, but not before unscrupulous clinics had managed to make a lot of money, and mess up a lot of heads.

Are fiber implants still being performed anyplace? We hope not—but beware. And don't consider any new method of putting hair on your head without first speaking to your family doctor.

A Better, Safer Way

Don't confuse the disastrous fiber implant method with a better, safer way. This is known as the cosmetic suture retainer process advocated by Maurice Mann of Hair Again, Ltd. in New York. It is quite different, and several well-trained, highly respected dermatologists in New York believe this method is an acceptable option for the individual who wants a full head of hair.

Maurice Mann describes it as more permanent than hairpieces or hair weaving (see Section Four), yet less radical than transplants. He introduced the concept in 1970, and proudly points to his own head as a living demonstration.

Mann decided that at twenty-five he was too young to be bald. He realized there were a lot of other people out there with the same problem—so making use of his own personal experience and his Harvard Business School training—he decided to do something about it.

He worked with physicians and technologists, and developed a system he describes as a cosmetic suture retainer process. Similar systems are available elsewhere.

What is the principle of this process?

Thin, soft surgical threads (called sutures) are placed by a physician in the fatty layers of tissues in the scalp; a technician later attaches small overlapping strips, or wefts of hair, to the sutures. These wefts are custom-made to match the person's existing hair. After all the wefts are attached, a stylist cuts and styles the hair so that it looks as natural as possible.

Stitches in your head? Won't this lead to the kind of problems that those fiber implants caused? Some critics worry that it will, yet thousands of men (and some women) have had many trouble-free years with this method.

The concept was invented by a bald-headed anesthesiologist. He initially made use of steel sutures with plastic coating, to which a wig was attached. This doesn't work out too well, because the wig creates tension on the steel loops and the skin can become chronically irritated and inflamed. Most physicians strongly advise against it.

The cosmetic suture retainer process is quite different. Strong nondissolving polypropelene sutures, like those used in heart surgery, are strategically placed in the scalp by a physician. He follows a "pattern" created by the stylist, who

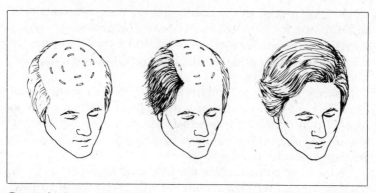

Cosmetic Suture Process
Surgical stitches are placed on the scalp, then wefts of hair are attached to the stitches, resulting in a full head of hair.

will attach the wefts of hair. These sutures can remain in the tissue of the scalp for a long period of time—safely.

How long is "a long period of time?"

According to Robert A. Berger, M.D., an assistant clinical professor of Dermatology at the Mount Sinai School of Medicine in New York, they can remain in place for years. However, men who are very athletic and put a great deal of stress on them may need to have some of them changed every twelve to eighteen months.

Dr. Berger's busy dermatology practice includes many patients who seek solutions to their hair loss. In addition to suture stitching, he offers them topical progesterone and minoxidil, transplants and reductions. He says, "The scalp is reasonably resistant to infection, and with reasonably good hygiene, the suture process offers a man who has fairly extensive baldness an opportunity to have a full head of hair."

Depending on the amount of baldness, twenty-five or more loop-shaped sutures are placed in the scalp, sometimes in areas between existing hair. It is a painless, quick procedure, which is done in the doctor's office. Dr. Berger, and some of the other physicians who do it, say that it takes about twenty minutes to complete about twenty-five stitches.

First they inject a local anesthetic into the scalp, then the stitches are placed in the predesignated areas. Patients take an antibiotic for a few days following the procedure. When they leave the doctor's office they return that same day to Hair Again, where the technician and stylist work together to create instant hair.

Maurice is quick to explain that they never cut off any of the existing hair, but simply add strips of synthetic hair to replace that which has been lost. After the hair is attached, a man can shower, shampoo his hair, swim, play tennis or anything else he wants.

There is, of course, some maintenance required.

His own hair will grow, and that will need careful cutting, but this can be done by any barber or stylist. The sutures may slightly loosen and migrate a bit, and will need to be replaced. The strips of hair need changing every two to three years, because they oxidize (turn a slightly red or yellow color) or otherwise seem to "wear out."

Thousands of men have had the process done at Hair Again, and probably many more at similar centers. Are they happy with it? For the most part, they seem to be. If at some time they change their mind, or are bothered by irritation, they can have the sutures removed. Scarring, if it takes place at all is minimal, according to Dr. Berger. Usually, after a few months the only visible evidence of removed sutures is a little dimpling, like an earring hole.

"But," he continues, "as a practical matter, it's not too great a problem because these men are usually eager to cover their baldness, and they will probably then opt for a hairpiece or weave."

Are there any medical complications other than the irritation mentioned? Critics of the procedure say that whenever a stitch is both inside the body *and* exposed to air, the potential for infection is high.

Theodor Kaufman, M.D., a Long Island, New York, surgeon who also does the procedure, feels that those critics probably have a skewed opinion of the process. Neither Dr. Kaufman nor Dr. Berger have seen any serious complications, although they admit that some people have local infections or soreness. "Frequently, it's because the person has been careless with basic scalp hygiene," says Dr. Berger.

Both agree that a man needs to be motivated and committed to the plan, because he will have to give his head more conscientious care than he did before. It is essential to keep both hair and stitches clean, and many men find that a hand-held shower head is great for getting at all the crevices.

The suture process itself is not very expensive, but it adds up quickly. The doctors bill the patients directly, and the usual fee is about $10 for each of the stitches. The custom-made hair, attached and styled, costs approximately another $2,000 at Hair Again. There are no regular maintenance costs other than the fees of your regular barber or stylist. When the hair needs changing, every three years or so, Hair Again charges only half of the original fee—approximately $1,000.

How does the suture retainer process look? It ranges from fair to excellent—and depends on many factors. Some colors look more natural than others, some men take better care of their hair, and some are so careless about it that the total effect is unnatural.

It is a good option for many people, and because the process is far more reversible than transplants—one that should be considered.

Tunnel Grafts

A professor of Dermatology at the University of British Columbia, Bernard J. Bendl, M.D., has published several articles in medical journals about a procedure, called the tunnel graft, which he describes as a secure, convenient, and safe way to attach a hairpiece. He says, "It is free of many of the complications of other attachments and is also reversible if the patient wishes to discontinue the technique."

Many surgeons do these tunnel grafts, also known as skin grafts, and usually they work closely with a hairpiece or wig manufacturer. Elliot Jacobs, M.D., prefers the tunnel grafts to the suture retainers. He feels they are safer, require less continuous care, and are unlikely to result in any complications.

Dr. Jacobs particularly recommends this procedure for people with advanced hair loss for whom only a complete hairpiece or wig will provide a significant amount of hair. Patients who are interested are often referred to him by Maurice Mann, the president of Hair Again, Ltd. According to Dr. Jacobs, "It is important that there be close cooperation between the surgeon and the hairpiece manufacturer, so as to achieve a precise fit."

How does the surgeon create a tunnel graft? Dr. Jacobs explains, "I take thin strips of skin from the area behind a person's lower abdomen and upper thigh (although some surgeons take skin from behind the ear) which I use to create three strong, skin-lined sturdy tunnels on the scalp, to serve as anchors for a hairpiece.

"This is an office procedure which is done under local anesthesia in about an hour and a half. I make two parallel incisions on the scalp at three sites—two in front, one in back. I then create a pocket or tunnel between the two parallel incisions underneath the scalp. Then I cut the graft I have removed from the groin into three pieces the size of postage stamps. (I stitch these grafts over little rubber tubes, to hold their shape.) With dissolving stitches, I sew the grafts to the edges of the incisions. After the three tunnels have healed, the rubber tubes are removed."

The hairpiece will later be held on the head by means of three small plastic clips. One side of each clip is inserted into each little tunnel, the other side is attached to the hairpiece.

After the surgery, little square dressings are placed on each graft. Some people temporarily wear a hairpiece, conventionally attached with tape, until the grafts are fully healed.

Recovery following graft surgery is uncomplicated. Any bleeding will respond to firm, steady pressure. Infections are prevented by oral antibiotics, and if do they occur, are easily treated. There may be swelling, but it should not be cause for any alarm. Care of the surgical sites on the groin and scalp is simple, and although strenuous physical activities have to

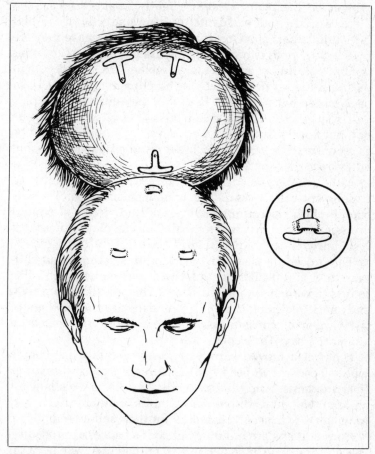

Tunnel Grafts with Hairpiece
Tunnel grafts are surgically placed on the scalp, to which a removable hairpiece with clips is securely attached.

be avoided for about two weeks after surgery, the procedure is not incapacitating.

Final healing takes place about six weeks after the surgery. The patient then begins to wear the hairpiece to which the clips are attached. These clips, inserted into the three strong tunnels on the scalp, create a slightly balanced tension. If there should be an accidental pull on one side of the hair piece, the other clips are driven in deeper because they are pointing in opposite directions. Precise placement of the clips is essential. If they are too close together, the hairpiece will pull and tug on the tunnels. If the clips are placed too far back on the hairpiece, the hairpiece may tend to pop up.

If someone pulls at the hairpiece, the clips might come out, but not the graft. Dr. Jacobs says, "The graft may not be as secure as your ear or nose, but it is quite safe for just about all average daily activities."

Although the procedure affords a certain sense of security, it does not offer twenty-four hour hair coverage. The wig should not be worn for sleeping, nor during very strenuous physical activities such as football. You can play tennis, wear hats, but you can't go swimming in it.

The procedure is equally good for men, women and children, and is especially popular with people who don't like to fuss too much with a hairpiece. "They can line it up right and put it on quickly, even in the dark. It relieves them of the burden of constantly wondering, 'Is my hairpiece on straight?'" says Dr. Jacobs.

It has also proved particularly welcome to those people whose heads have been badly scarred by those disastrous fiber implants. And, as Dr. Bendl says, "It is excellent for children who have suffered from burns or other trauma, and to whom a hairpiece is essential for their self-esteem."

Tunnel grafts are a minor but serious surgical procedure that must be done by someone well trained in how to perform them. Like most of the surgical procedures we have discussed, tunnel grafts are not covered by insurance, unless there is medical cause for the hair loss. The cost of the surgery is around $1,200, and the hairpieces range in price from $350 to $750 or more. As discussed in chapter 8, hairpieces must be replaced from time to time, and do require care and upkeep.

Tunnel grafts, like transplants, flaps, and the cosmetic surgery suture process, are an option that is well worth exploring. When the procedure is done properly it is a very satisfactory way to get almost-instant hair.

Unlike transplants, tunnel grafts are easily reversible, requiring only a minor surgical procedure to remove the grafts. Three H-shaped scars will result, which are less visible than the scars remaining after the removal of stitches in the suture retainer process.

It would be wise, before deciding on a suture retainer or on tunnel grafts, to wear a hairpiece or wig for six months or a year. Be sure you like the way it looks and feels, and that you really want the added sense of security the procedure will give. You may find yourself perfectly happy wearing the wig without it. Hairpieces and wigs are better than they were in the past, and in the next chapter we will discuss the various types that are available.

Putting It Back: Cosmetically

CHAPTER 8

Hairpieces
and Wigs

THEY DON'T CALL THEM RUGS ANYMORE. OR EVEN TOUPEES. THEY
don't attach them with irritating carpet tape, and they're not
heavy and hot. Most of the time people can't even tell you're
wearing one. Unfortunately, when people think about hairpieces they conjure up images of their Uncle Joe nervously
patting his head, his dark red hairpiece perched atop his gray
sideburns. They remember how it always set them to gig-
gling.

But Ricardo Montalban, Burt Reynolds, William Shatner,
Jack Klugman and maybe the guy next door all wear them.
No one *has* to look like Uncle Joe.

Hairpieces are better and more natural than ever before,
but these improvements cost money. You can't just go into a
store and buy a hairpiece like you would a new pair of shoes.
Sure, hairpieces come in different sizes, shapes and colors,
and you probably could get something that would fit, but it
wouldn't look very good.

Whether your hair loss is from pattern baldness or any
other cause, is temporary or permanent, it *is* possible to put
it back naturally and attractively. But you have to go about
it in the right way.

In many communities there are custom hairpiece designers who can make a hairpiece for you. Often local barbers or
hairstylists can order these custom pieces and then do some

final touches. They also maintain them for you. Or you may
be able to order a hairpiece directly from a designer by mail.
There are also some firms that adjust various stock items to
fit your personal measurements, a procedure which can
sometimes work out quite satisfactorily.

Does He or Doesn't He?

I used to think I could spot a hairpiece thirty feet away. So,
you can imagine my surprise when waiting on line to get my
photograph taken for a driver's license, I saw the middle-
aged man in front of me take off his hair before he posed for
his picture.

I was intrigued, and while the rest of the people on the
line stood there with their mouths open, I asked him, "Why
in the world did you do that?"

He explained: he's a salesman who feels a hairpiece en-
hances his appearance and ability to make sales. But when
he's relaxing at home on weekends he doesn't wear it, so he
thought it better to be "au naturel" on his driver's license.

This encounter led me to reassess my hairpiece acumen.
I realized that, like all of us, I was good at recognizing the
obvious. If a hairpiece is obvious, it's because it doesn't look
genuine. The good ones are so natural we don't think about
them. Unless someone tells us.

Tell the truth now. Would you be able to tell that Burt
Reynolds had a hairpiece, if you didn't know he wore one?
I wouldn't.

Natural-Looking Hairpieces

For any number of reasons, it is easier to make a woman's
hairpiece or wig look natural. On pages 129–31 we will
discuss women's wigs, but now, let us focus on what makes
a man's hairpiece look natural.

A hairpiece must reflect a man's age, complexion and life
style. If it doesn't, it will stick out like a sore thumb. There
is a great temptation to try to turn back the clock and wear
your hair dark and abundantly luxurious. Resist it. It will

not look natural. While a woman can sometimes realize her fantasies with an unusual or very full wig, a man who does that invariably looks foolish, and sometimes even older.

If you look at the advertisements in the Yellow Pages, magazines, or newspapers under "Hair Replacement," you will notice that "nondetectable," "natural," and "fine quality" are the buzzwords of the industry.

And they should be.

Who Should Wear a Hairpiece?

Anyone who wants to cover up hair loss should consider wearing a hairpiece. You don't have to wait until you've lost a lot of hair, since you can have a very small, partial piece if that's all you need. Actually, if you begin to wear a hairpiece when you first start to bald, friends and coworkers may not even notice the difference. As hair loss increases (if it does), you can continue to get additional coverage.

If you are considering one of the surgical/cosmetic approaches discussed in the last chapter (suture process or tunnel graft) you should wear a hairpiece and get used to it *before* you undergo the surgery. If you are unhappy with the hairpiece, you have only spent some money. If you do anything surgical you will have to "undo" it should you change your mind.

Making the Decision

Do not buy a hairpiece in haste. You will only regret it. Having made a significant dent in your wallet, it will mock you from the closet.

The House of Louis Feder in New York has been making men's top-of-the-line hairpieces for over sixty-five years. Jerry Roman, the general manager, explains that a good hairpiece should make you look the way you would if you hadn't lost your hair. He says, "The hair should flow just like your own, and appear to grow from the scalp."

Charles Alfieri of New York, another top-notch hairpiece maker, concurs. "The most important thing is the hairline.

If that doesn't look natural, nothing will. But we also have to consider balance. Whatever we're going to put on top of the head should be in balance with the sides and the back. If the sides are fine or thin, we can't give a man a lot of hair or it will overpower him. He will have to have a slightly receding, light hairline.

"We want to make a fifty year old man look forty-five or fifty, not twenty or twenty-five," Alfieri says.

If you want to have hair enough to look like the "you that would have been" and you are willing to devote the time and money needed to make it look natural, then a hairpiece may be just the thing for you.

A Good Hairpiece

What makes a good hairpiece? A hairpiece is good if it looks natural and feels comfortable.

It will look natural
• if the hairline and color are appropriate to your age.
• if the color matches your sideburns and fringe hair.
• if you can't see where the hairpiece ends and your hair begins.
• if the hair looks like "real" hair.
It will feel comfortable
• if is lightweight—no more than a couple of ounces.
• if it isn't hot.
• if it properly adheres to your head.

All of the pros agree on these points—but there are different approaches.

The First Step

Once you have made the decision, you should visit a good full-service salon, where the consultant will talk with you to get a sense of your lifestyle, thoughts and needs. He (the consultant doesn't have to be a he, but usually is) will probably show you some illustrations or photographs so that you can get a sense of what might be suitable for you.

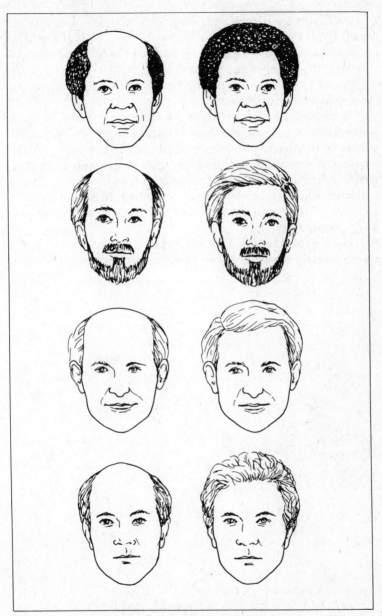

Hairpieces: Before and After

At Charles Alfieri's your hair will be washed, and then the blender (a person, not a food processor) will come in to see you. Samples of hair are taken from the back temple and crown (if you have any there) enabling Alfieri to assess the correct color hair for the hairpiece. A few different shades are custom blended to match the precise color and texture of your own hair. If a man has a little gray in the temples and a little less gray in the back, a third color is used for the front of the hairpiece, usually a mix of the temple and back colors. If a man doesn't have any gray in his remaining hair, Alfieri highlights the front so as to soften the look. Since a hairpiece will not hide your existing hair, it is vital that the match be right and that there is a natural unbroken line at any overlapping areas.

Then someone will take careful measurements and make a pattern for the foundation of your hairpiece.

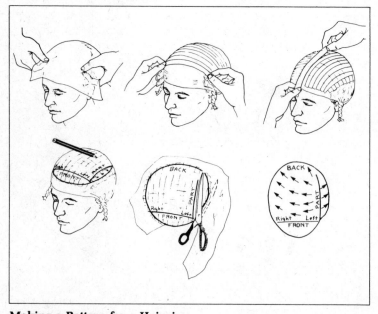

Making a Pattern for a Hairpiece
A pattern is carefully made of the man's head before the hairpiece is made.

The Foundation

What gave hairpieces their negative image years ago were those heavy, uncomfortable, helmetlike foundations made of cotton or rubber. Today's foundations are made of lightweight sheer materials, often synthetic, which are strong but comfortable.

Alfieri uses a nylon base, sort of a fishing twine material, which is strong, lightweight and "shampooable." Roman likes a durable base of nylon (a preshrunk type of material similar to umbrellas) and silk. He says it gives his hairpieces great durability. Lace bases are very lightweight, but Roman doesn't recommend lace to anyone who is going to give the hairpiece a lot of hard wear. It is also very expensive because the material is imported from France. But it is, he says, "the ultimate."

Ben Z. Kaplan has been in the hair replacement business a long time, and has seen everything. And he believes many hairpieces are overpriced. He describes his Universal Winners, Inc. as the world's first complete department store for men's hairpiece needs. He sells them directly to consumers, and through barber shops and salons throughout the country.

Kaplan feels that lace is impractical, and is very satisfied with the durable flesh-colored fabric or transparent monofilament bases he uses. He also makes an ultra-thin monofilament which he describes as similar to those of Alfieri, Roman and other high-priced custom designers. Kaplan's are generally mass produced (but by hand) and come in various sizes, such as five by seven, six by eight and seven by nine.

Human or Synthetic?

"Only natural European hair can be used," one expert says.

"Synthetic hair holds the shape and color better," says another.

"A mixture of human and synthetic hair works very well," some say.

"Never mix human and synthetic hair," state some pros.

"Yak (goat) hair is perfect for the grays and whites," many people agree.

Harvey Russo, who custom designs wonderfully natural-looking hairpieces for Top Priority in New York, imports hair from the mountains of Italy, and thinks, "Italian women have the finest hair. They don't use dyes or hairspray and there's very little pollution in the mountains. Their hair is fresh and natural so it maintains its shine and body much longer than any other hair."

Jerry Roman and Charles Alfieri also prefer Italian and other European hair. It can be stripped of color and then dyed with a good fabric dye to match a man's own natural or dyed hair. Because all hair, including synthetic hair, oxidizes, it is important to be able to restore color. They say synthetic hair doesn't dye as well, which is one reason human hair is superior.

Alfieri doesn't like to mix human and synthetic hair in one piece because they have to be treated differently. He explains, "You use rollers to put a curl or wave in hair. You would then apply a chemical to the human hair, but shoot steam into the synthetic hair. If you combine both kinds of hair in one hairpiece you have a problem."

Alfieri and Roman use synthetic hair for pieces made especially for swiming, tennis, boating and other sports activities. These hairpieces aren't as natural looking as the human hairpieces, but when wet, the synthetic don't tangle or mat like human hair, and they dry considerably faster. These synthetic hairpieces, both men agree, are fine for casual wearing, but don't look right in the board room.

Kaplan feels that synthetic hair is superior to human. He says that so little is used in each hairpiece that the price differential is inconsequential, so he doesn't base his decision on cost. "The early synthetics were really bad and looked somewhat like 'mannequin' hair. But now they are terrific. Synthetic hair doesn't fade and oxidize as much as human hair does, and it blends better too."

On one issue there was agreement even among those who uphold the doctrine of human hair only: it's almost impossible to get white human hair or to prevent oxidization if they do get it—so they use yak hair to blend in the light grays and whites.

Putting It All Together

When hair blend, foundation fit and contour, workmanship and styling all come together to make a hairpiece that's natural looking, it can fool anyone.

As the foundation rests comfortably on a form in the workroom, experienced workers, by hand, attach one strand of hair at a time. The hairline in particular must be carefully worked to provide the "trompe l'oeil" which constitutes a good hairpiece.

Ideally, wig hair should interlock, blending imperceptibly with your own hair but not covering it. "Sometimes, if his own hair is very fine, and he has a broad face and needs a little more hair, we will cover some of it," says Alfieri.

After the hairpiece has been constructed, the styling process begins. A "prestyling" is done even before the client returns. When he comes back, six to eight weeks later, the

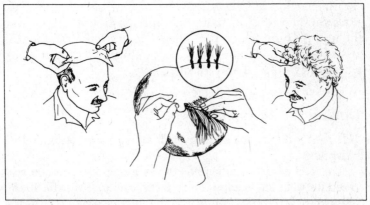

Making a Hairpiece
A foundation is cut according to the pattern, and then the hair is attached by hand. Final styling is done after the hairpiece is completed.

hairpiece is put on his head so the stylist can do final touches. The client gets instructions on how to wear and care for it, and is given a head form to keep it on overnight. Then he is on his way.

Keeping It on Your Head

Remember that old slapstick comedy where the fellow chases his hairpiece across a windy street?

Actually, it's not something you have to worry about because a properly fitting hairpiece is easily and comfortably affixed to the head. Ben Kaplan says that one of the questions most often asked by customers is, "What is the best adhesive?"

He replies that no one single adhesive is best for everybody. Universal offers a variety of tapes, some so strong that a person could swim, sleep or engage in "intimate" activities without fear of the hairpiece coming loose. They also sell spray, brush and roll-on adhesives as well as the old standby, spirit gum.

All the experts recommend contoured and curved hypoallergenic, double-faced, adhesive transparent tapes. Tapes should be changed every few days, but some people get an extra few days out of them by applying liquid adhesive to the top. A comb which fits into the man's remaining hair is also often sewn into the hairpieces. Alfieri uses a comb-clip which snaps closed and locks.

Caring for Your Hairpiece

"Please," all our experts say, "don't sleep or shower in a hairpiece."

There is general agreement that a hairpiece must be well cared for to keep its good looks. Jerry Roman gives his clients precise instructions on putting the hairpiece on their heads. First, of course, he tells them to apply the tape to the designated area.

"Then with your right hand holding the front of the hairpiece and your left hand securing the back, place the hair-piece gently on your head. The center portion of the hairpiece should be directly in line with your nose. Check in the mirror, and press down on all portions of the hairpiece for a thirty second period. Then, using a wide-tooth comb or fine-bristle brush, comb the hair as if it were your own. A quick spray of lanolin and hairspray will have you all set to meet the world. And it takes no longer than putting on your tie.

"Remove it gently by moistening a piece of cloth with adhesive remover and gently placing cloth between scalp and hairpiece base. Gradually start lifting it—never pull or rip off the hairpiece. Then comb it gently and put it on the head form."

Jerry Roman and Harvey Russo recommend that a hair-piece be professionally cleaned every three or four weeks, although you *can* clean it at home. House of Feder even sells a "quick dry" hairpiece cleaner.

Many of Charles Alfieri's clients come in regularly to have their hairpiece "serviced," which means cleaned, brushed and checked over. At the same time they have their own hair cut. But Alfieri feels you can do a good job of washing your own hairpiece, if you wish. Since his pieces are all made on a synthetic base, they are truly wash and wear.

"Just lay the hairpiece in the sink, wet it, place a nice mild shampoo on it, and massage it like it's your own head, using a soft little nail brush. Then pick the hairpiece up in your hands and run it underneath the faucet to wash off the soap. Gently squeeze the water off it, roll it up in a towel, put it on the head form overnight, or dry it with the blow dryer. It won't lose its shape," he says.

Hairpieces eventually change color and oxidize (espe-cially in summer), and need to be redyed. The fabric dyes work well on them, and although most of our experts say it's not a do-it-yourself project, Universal sells color restorers for faded pieces—in keeping with their philosophy that it doesn't have to cost a fortune to buy or maintain a hairpiece.

Good and loving care of your hairpiece will extend its life, and help to make it look its best. Still, even the best cared for hairpiece will need replacement from time to time.

How Long Will It Last?

All my experts say that the most you can get out of a hair-piece—human or synthetic—is a few years. After all, our own hair doesn't last indefinitely (remember all that information about anagen and telogen hairs, and natural shedding), and so I began to wonder. Perhaps those artificial looking hairpieces I see when I'm waiting on line for a bus or movie (where I quietly count the heads of potential readers for this book!) aren't all the result of shoddy workmanship. They've just seen their better days.

Depending on the "wear and tear" you give your hairpiece, and the kind of base chosen, you can expect to get anywhere from a year and a half to four years from a hairpiece. This is especially true if you have two. Most of those who make them, and those who wear them, agree that a man should have more than one hairpiece just in case.

Imagine what it was like one day last summer for my neighbor Paul. He has been wearing a hairpiece (no, not the same one) for twenty-five years, and the only time he takes it off is when he's putting out the garbage.

One rush hour, in the midst of a heat wave, Paul was standing on a subway platform. He loosened his tie and, you guessed it, to get a little air on his scalp, he released the tape on the front of his hairpiece. As the train came roaring down the track Paul was pushed and shoved, and he stood in shock as he watched his beautiful new hairpiece go right over the side of the platform, onto the tracks. It wasn't until the tracks were cleaned that night that Paul's hairpiece was rescued. Before the "lost and found" department would hand it over to him they wanted proof it was his. Paul felt a little like Cinderella, but the hairpiece fit him so well that even the tough-minded New York City Transit Authority was convinced he was the rightful owner.

Such accidents are rare indeed, but the man who gets caught in a rainstorm when he's planned a night on the town, or is heading to a PTA meeting, should, according to Jerry Roman, have an extra hairpiece so he doesn't have to put himself "on hold."

Alfieri doesn't feel it's a necessity. A man can restore a hairpiece himself in no time at all, he says, and the sports hairpiece can always do in a pinch. "But," he adds, "a lot of men agree they feel 'safer' knowing they always have a spare."

Everyone agrees that if a man has two hairpieces they will simply last twice as long. So why have only one?

Can I Afford It?

You can get a hairpiece for as little as $100. It probably won't look natural or be terribly comfortable. But it will last. Because you won't wear it much.

A good hairpiece isn't cheap. Cost is based on several factors: type of base, quality of hair, size of area that is being covered, and workmanship. A good hairpiece from House of Feder, Charles Alfieri or Top Priority can cost anywhere from $400 to well over $1,000. These men say one of the keys to their success is the personal quality control they exert over their workrooms. Their craftspeople are well trained, take an interest in the finished product, and often look on proudly when a man walks out in the hairpiece they have made.

But Kaplan stands by his modestly priced stock hairpieces, saying they look "custom made", because some are, and others are individualized and adjusted. In his own $500 hairpiece, Ben Kaplan looks natural and comfortable. He says that many of the pieces he sells to barbers for only a few hundred dollars are the same as those sold elsewhere for $1,000.

When a barber tells you he will have your hairpiece made for you, it's sometimes hard to know if he is dealing with a custom-made salon where the hairpieces are made on the premises, or from a wholesaler/retailer who imports stock pieces from Hong Kong and Korea. You may get a fair price, but you may also end up paying $1,000 for Kaplan's $250 piece. Or you may get it for $350. Depends on your barber.

The old saying "You pay for what you get" doesn't always hold true here. Or does it?

Many men are willing to pay for the confidence they gain from being serviced in a comfortable, relaxed, total-care hair salon. Their own hair is cared for, their hairpiece is made with loving hands (they can meet the people in the back workrooms and see it "growing"), and it is cleaned and cared for on the premises. They know they won't be allowed out of the place unless they look right. So they feel the attention they get is well worth the money. For a monthly service visit to House of Feder, Charles Alfieri or Top Priority, the cost is about $20. No more than it would cost if you had your own hair and went to a good stylist.

Medical insurance will only pay for a hairpiece if it is a replacement for hair lost through an accident or illness. Actors and models can usually take it as a tax deduction, but salesman can't. It's worth discussing with your accountant.

If you are considering a hairpiece, remember:
- A hairpiece is only as good as the hands that make it, so all the experts say.
- Custom-made hairpieces are more expensive than individualized stock pieces; human hair costs more than synthetic hair.
- The lighter weight foundations or bases give a more natural look, but are costlier and less durable than the stronger, heavier ones.
- A hairpiece must be right for you, appropriate to your age, coloring and facial features as well as to your lifestyle. Only if it looks natural and feels comfortable will you be happy in it.
- The professional hairpiece stylist makes sure it "all comes together" and he instructs you in its care.

A good hairpiece can be viewed simply as a fashion accessory, or as an integral part of your everyday appearance. It can be next-best to having your own hair. Some men claim it is every bit as good as growing it back or surgically putting it back, and won't consider any other way of replacing lost hair. Others see it as a temporary means only, and want something more permanent. Still others say that the chief drawback is the fact that they can't wear it twenty-four hours a day, and sooner or later someone will have to see them without hair. Single men don't know how to tell a new date, and fathers sometimes say that they feel awkward in front of their children. And children are embarrassed when their friends find out. For these reasons the hair weaving concept described in the next chapter is worth considering.

Men's Wigs

Men sometimes decide to get a wig, rather than a hairpiece, because the "look" they have in mind doesn't blend with their own sideburns or fringe hair. But more often, a man wears a wig because he has no sideburns or fringe hair. Temporary or permanent hair loss from accidents or illness (see chapter ten for information on the effects of chemotherapy and radiation) may include the loss of sideburns and fringe hair. Then only a wig will suffice.

A bad wig can look dreadful. Too much hair, and unnatural sideburns on anyone past puberty will result in a eunuchlike look. Thus, men's wigs must be carefully made. The foundation must fit perfectly. And sideburns must be attached to a very lightweight, transparent base if they are to look natural.

A good custom-made wig can look fine, but it will cost anywhere from $1,400 up. If it is truly a prosthesis, that is, a medical replacement for a missing piece of the body, many health insurance companies will help pay for it, or you can take it as a medical tax deduction.

Women's Wigs

Women wear wigs for many reasons. To look different, to save the time and trouble of getting their hair just right, and to save money. Yes, save money. Because a natural-looking synthetic wig can cost less than weekly visits to a beauty salon.

But many women wear wigs because they have little choice. Their hair loss, temporary or permanent, is pronounced, and they are miserable. A man who chooses to bare his crown has plenty of company. A woman looks terrible and she knows it. A wig will let her look like her former self.

If your hair is irreversibly lost, or is taking its time to grow back, where do you turn?

Frequently your beauty parlor may sells wigs or can get one for you. You can go to a wig salon, such as Joseph Fleischer, which is under the ownership of The House of Feder. Department stores also sell wigs, but most market them as "fashion accessories," because they do not wish to associate them with hair loss.

More than seven million women's wigs are imported into the United States each year, and approximately a million of those are distributed by Eva Gabor, International. Ken Roper, Jr., vice-president of marketing, explains that their wigs are made of a monocrylic fiber with "excellent memory qualities," which means they don't lose their curl. He pointed out the advances the industry has made in these synthetics— even the blue-blacks no longer have that shiny, artificial color that once was the hallmark of a synthetic wig.

These ready-to-wear wigs, as they are called, are just that. There is such a variety of styles and colors that just about any woman can find a wig that is "her." They are comfortable and cool, and easy to wash with a mild baby shampoo. Although most are mass produced, some styles are hand-made. Ken Roper says that many of the salons who sell their wigs add a lace front, to which they attach some extra hair, to give it an even more natural look. Other manufacturers also sell stock wigs, and these too can be individually customized by beauty parlors or wig stores.

Gabor wigs, like other ready-to-wear wigs, often cost less than $50. Sometimes, a department store will have a two-for-the-price-of-one special, bringing the cost below the price of a hat.

How long do these wigs last? Ken Roper says that if a woman uses a wig constantly, she will need two. And they will probably need yearly replacement.

Nothing but the real thing will do for some women. They want human hair, and they want to feel that it is made especially for them. The colors are better blended and more natural looking, and the hair has a softer look, but the wig will need a great deal more maintenance. Such a wig can be purchased through beauty salons or at wig stores.

At Joseph Fleischer, the women's wigs are made with the same custom attention given to the men's hairpieces.

Women's wigs last longer than men's hairpieces, according to the folks at Joseph Fleischer, even if worn daily. Why? Perhaps women are more careful with them. But in all probability it is because they don't wear them around the house, or while cooking. Some men never take off their hairpieces except to shower or sleep.

Costs of women's wigs range widely, depending on several factors such as materials, amount of hair and stylists. At Fleischer, natural Italian hair wigs run from $1,400 to $2,500, but may last up to seven or eight years. The price of a wig that is a blend of human and synthetic hair, which minimizes oxidation, is between $1,000 and $1,500. One of these should last up to ten years. An all handmade synthetic wig lasts about two years, and costs between $350 and $550.

Joseph Fleischer recommends that their wigs be cleaned and serviced by them, but some beauty salons are able to do it.

If you are considering a wig, remember:
• Shop carefully.
• Avoid design and color inappropriate to your age and coloring.
• A bare head or a hat will look better than an ill-fitting wig.
• If you have two wigs, don't worry if they are not exactly the same. Even your own hair can look a little different each day.

CHAPTER 9

Hair Weaves, Fusion and Extensions

HAIR WEAVES, FUSION AND EXTENSIONS ARE CLEVER IDEAS. Instead of being attached to the *scalp* surgically or with adhesive, the replacement hair is attached to *hair* itself.

The concept is fine, but, unfortunately, its execution is sometimes far from fine. It can, in the hands of the wrong people, damage your own hair and cause hair loss.

Weaving, fusion, and some of the more sophisticated extension techniques are often lumped together, so it is important that we discuss each technique individually and note the major differences.

Hair Weaving

Hair weaving has been around for a long time. It was originally designed and brought over to this country by blacks. Weaving usually begins by braiding the person's own hair very tightly across the head. Additional hair, in wefts, is then attached and anchored to this hair. Weaving is practiced by many salons or individuals as a fashion concept rather than as a replacement for hair loss.

Hair weaves for men are usually designed for hair loss, and often make use of a net base which is anchored to the remaining hair, and to which the wefts of hair are then sewn.

The major disadvantages of hair weaving are that it makes thorough washing of the scalp very difficult, and that it can cause permanent traction alopecia in people whose hair loss might only have been temporary, or who might not even have suffered hair loss prior to the weave.

The cosmetic result is not consistently good for everyone. There is a somewhat flat appearance. And a great deal of hair spray is required to keep it in place. There is little or no movement to the hair, which may be acceptable with curly or kinky hair but is artificial looking when the hair is straight. The straight hair is usually overlapped like the shingles on a roof, and when the wind blows in the opposite direction, your hair may resemble the sail on a boat. Also when the wind blows in the wrong direction the scalp looks like lines of railroad tracks.

Hair weaving offers an interesting cosmetic variation for women. It can be very satisfactory as a temporary plan, perhaps for a special occasion or a holiday period. If you wish to keep a weave permanently it will have to be reapplied often, because your own hair continues to grow, loosening the weave.

Weaving has its aesthetic limitations, and most dermatologists do not recommend it as a regular method of hair replacement, particularly because of the difficulties in keeping the scalp clean and the potential for traction alopecia.

Hair Fusion

Hair fusion is a process by which synthetic or human hair is linked with your own hair using a water insoluble, often caustic glue that forms a chemical bond with the hair. The appearance is often satisfactory but most dermatologists caution against it. They say the strong chemicals which are used to link and later remove the hair can lead to scalp irritations and mild to severe allergic reactions. Profuse hair breaking as well as traction alopecia can also develop, and the same problems of scalp hygiene exist with this method as with the hair weave.

Hair Extensions

An interesting concept in hair replacement is a sophisticated form of hair weaving, often called hair extension. Popularized by The Hair Club for Men, Ltd., with several branches in the New York metropolitan area, Boston, San Francisco, Los Angeles, Houston, Fort Lauderdale, Florida, Connecticut and Toronto, and more on the horizon, and by other stylists throughout the country—it is worn by a variety of extremely active, image-conscious men (and women too) who want to have twenty-four hour trouble-free hair.

Extension is often confused with hair weaving but differs in several respects. With the extension method, the hair is attached to a lightweight base in single strands rather than wefts. The base or matrix is attached to the person's own hair and the replacement hair combines with the existing scalp hair to form natural, free movement. It is permanent, but easily reversible, and when done by well trained and experienced technicians at reputable, professional salons, should not cause any problems.

Who Should Consider Hair Extension?

Men whose hair loss has resulted from pattern baldness are excellent candidates for hair extension. According to Sy Sperling, president of Hair Club for Men, Ltd., it is very effective in those men whose fringe and side hair are healthy. Evan Miller, executive vice-president of the firm, and founder of Hair Images, a similar firm which has recently been acquired by Hair Club, adds, "I believe that a woman should have an extension only if her hair loss is from pattern baldness, or if she has an area of permanent loss due to a congenital condition or scarring. If her side and back hair isn't strong, it could be further weakened by the extension, and thus has the potential to be lost. I would recommend she have a full medical evaluation, and then perhaps consider getting a wig."

Both men state that a reputable firm should select their

clients carefully, and often will turn someone down or tell them to wait a while, if their hair loss is very slight. If the loss appears to stem from a condition which can be medically corrected, they recommend the client see a physician.

Many of the men who come in for a consultation have had transplants and are unhappy with the results. Sperling says, "I've seen a lot of good transplants, but they do have their limitations. Sometimes the doctor tells a man, 'we just can't do anymore,' so he comes to us because he wants a full head of hair. We make good use of his transplanted hair, blending it in with our system for a really fine looking frontal hairline."

Men who have had hairpieces, or women who have had wigs, often opt for hair extension because they are unhappy with any system which they have to remove to sleep or shower. Some people don't want anyone—ever—to see them without hair.

Many clients and their friends feel that hair extension offers a natural looking appearance, unmatched by any other form of hair replacement.

Making the Decision

Hair extension as practiced at the Hair Club for Men, where it is described as a "Strand-by-Strand®" hair system, requires an ongoing commitment from the client.

Here's why. After it's done, you can't just wash your hair one-two-three, in a haphazard fashion. You must also be willing to spend the time and money to return to the salon every six to eight weeks to have the hair tightened and the entire system serviced. And every two or three years you must have it all replaced. You can't just send your hair replacement in by messenger or by mail as you can do with a hairpiece. A man who travels for months at a time, or whose trips are lengthy and unpredictable, or who lives far from an extension center and can't get there on a regular basis, may find hair extension is not for him.

But if you *can* give the time and money to it, have some hair with which to work, and want a full head of hair—you should seriously consider this excellent method.

The First Step

The first step is a consultation at a salon that does a good hair extension method. There are some individual and subtle differences, but generally, at the first visit, the consultant talks with you to determine the look you are trying to achieve. There is an almost unlimited number of hairstyles that you can have, although the short, conservative look is probably the hardest to achieve. It is also possible to dye and/or permanent your own hair before the new hair is added. This will be considered at the initial consultation.

An accurate pattern is made of your head, and samples of your hair are taken in order to match color and texture. In about six weeks you return to have the system placed on your head.

During the period while you are awaiting your new hair, the salon prepares a lightweight, transparent porous grid or template to conform exactly to the shape of your head.

Sperling explains that they have developed a new filament grid, unique to Hair Club, which is so thin as to be even more undetectable to the touch or eye than was ever before possible. Into this grid, individual strands of hair are added, one at a time. This hair is matched to your own hair for density, direction of hair flow, wave pattern, and of course color. And, according to your specific needs, some of these holes in the grid are left open, so that if your hair loss is not extensive, your own hair can be pulled through. For this reason, anyone, from those whose hair is thinning or slightly balding to those who are really bald, can make good use of the system.

Getting Your New Hair

When the system is ready, you come back to the salon for the second visit. In many styling centers a very strong, but fine nylon fiber is worked into the hair around your thinning area and pulled taut. The grid is then attached to this braid-like combination of hair and fiber.

But Hair Club for Men has even found a way to eliminate this braid. Light weight, thin retainer wires are built into the perimeters of the grid, and the person's own hair goes through these retainer wires and locks into place with an innovative, secure device. This new technology permits adjustable tension, better drainage and is faster to attach and service. Your replacement hair will blend imperceptibly with your own back and side hair.

A stylist then gives you a final cutting and shaping, and instructions on how to care for your new hair. A couple of hours after you came through the door, you are on your way with a head full of hair.

Human or Synthetic?

Most hair extension practitioners use human hair. "Our clients are out there in the sun, rain, and wind, and they sleep and shower wearing their system, so it's got to stand up to all that, and still last a couple of years. We have to use the best hair, and know that if it oxidizes we can successfully dye it back to its original color. Synthetic or even second-rate human hair just won't do for us," says Miller.

Sperling says that they have developed a process that minimizes the problems with oxidation of natural hair.

Sperling, like a proud school kid with his new science project, says to me, "Go ahead, run your hand through my hair—would you know it wasn't all my own growing hair?"

I had to admit he could have fooled me.

Care of Hair at Home

If you follow the simple directions you are given, you will probably find the system trouble-free. Those people who have had problems with the hair extension method usually are careless about hygiene.

Clients are advised to wait a few days, or even a week after the installation of the system before washing their hair, in order to allow natural scalp oils to work into it. The system also needs to loosen up just a bit so that you can thoroughly wash and rinse the scalp through the grid, and avoid any soap build-up.

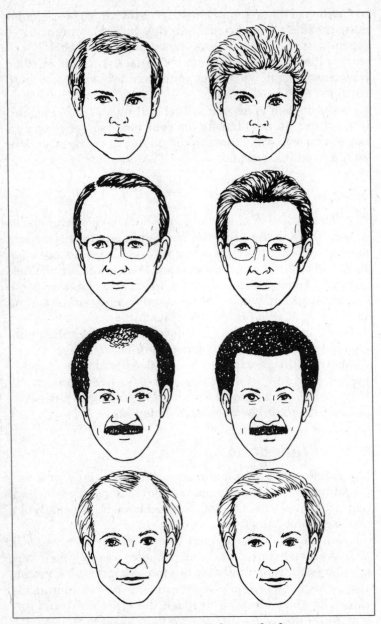

Hair Extensions: Before and After

Gentle but thorough brushing, frequent washing (vital for the care of scalp and hair), and drying with a towel and a portable hand-held dryer is all the care that should be needed.

"A man who has had a problem with dandruff can still have this system," says Sy Sperling, "but he will have to wash his hair frequently, and extremely thoroughly, because he will be more vulnerable to the dandruff."

Everyone, however, must rinse the hair and scalp through the matrix. A good shower spray or nozzle that can remove all suds and bacteria and prevents build-up of residue, is a wise investment.

Maintenance of the System

A drawback to the hair extension systems are the mandatory maintenance sessions that are needed on a regular basis. Your own hair will continue to grow (yes, even that fringe hair grows), and the system will naturally loosen. So periodically you must return to the salon to have the system readjusted and have your own hair cut.

Depending on the rate at which your hair grows, this maintenance may be necessary anywhere from every six to eight weeks. I met clients who come in every six weeks, and who looked as well before as after their maintenance session.

During the hour or hour-and-a-half that you are there, your own hair is washed, the replacement hair is professionally cleaned and carefully checked to see if it needs any repairs, and the system is then put back into place.

Evan Miller suggests that even though these return visits are usually perceived as a disadvantage, they can be turned into a benefit. At the salon you get a good haircut, the hair is resnugged within yours, and you go out the door looking just right. Twelve months of the year, twenty-four hours a day, a man with an extension system looks his very best— as opposed to a man who might buy an excellent hairpiece but not continue to have it properly serviced. Hair extension clients have no choice: they must have the system professionally serviced or give it up.

Although the system presents time juggling for the man

who travels a lot or lives outside the city where it was made—
there is still hope. There are many excellent firms throughout
the country to which Sperling, Miller and others can refer
you for ongoing service, or for an occasional appointment
when you are traveling.

Approximately every three years the entire system needs
to be replaced because the extension hair loses its vitality,
becomes brittle, and just generally deteriorates.

Does S/He or Doesn't S/He?

When hair extension is done right, it is next to impossible
to know a person has it. People from all walks of life—
entertainers, executives, salespeople, and professional ath-
letes are happy with it.

Does the hair separate and show the tell-tale grid? Does it
look strange blowing in the wind? No. It looks natural—and
you really can't tell a person is wearing it unless you put
your hand firmly on the top of the head. Then you can feel
a slight ridge that is the "give-away." Even this is almost
undetectable with Hair Club's new method.

What about water sports? Will you look strange coming
up from a dive, or when the sea breezes run through your
hair while waterskiing?

Ask a marathon swimmer who has the system. He has
swum around Manhattan Island and the English Channel and
practices in a pool regularly. As he stepped out of New York
City's Hudson River, the television cameras focused closely
on his face and head. I never would have guessed it wasn't
his hair. The chlorine and other chemicals take their toll, so
he has his entire system changed yearly. But it looks fine—
wet or dry.

Costs

There's no question about it. The cost of the hair extension
system is the greatest disadvantage. It is expensive. And unlike transplants or hair flaps, it is not a one-time expense.

Depending on the amount of hair that has to be replaced,

and on which of the many salons in the country you choose, the initial cost has a wide range: $1,000–$4,000. A tremendous discount is given if a second system is ordered, and the replacement system three years later is often at half-price or less. The regular maintenance sessions are approximately $50.

If the system is installed to conceal an area of scarring alopecia due to a congenital condition, an accident or other trauma, medical insurance may contribute towards the costs. Actors and models may be able to take a tax deduction.

A Quick Review

If you are considering a hair weave, fusion, or extension, carefully weigh the plus against the minus. Hair weaving in its basic form serves a purpose, but many critics feel that it can cause traction alopecia and is not a good ongoing system of hair replacement. Hair fusion is unsatisfactory, sometimes resulting in further hair loss. Hair extension, which some people lump together with hair weaving, is far better than the original concept from which it developed.

It looks and feels natural, affords a man a full head of youthful hair, and is easy to maintain on a daily basis. However, it has two distinct disadvantages. The initial cost is high, and professional maintenance is necessary, involving further time and expense. Before having an extension system installed on your head, call your local Better Business Bureau to be sure that complaints have not been registered against the facility, and speak with other people whom they have serviced. Remember, the method, no matter how technically sophisticated, is only as good as the operators who perform it. At Hair Club for Men, and other responsible facilities, operators are careful not to place undue stress on the remaining hair.

If you want abundant twenty-four-hour hair—instantly— hair extension is a method you should certainly consider.

SECTION FIVE

Special Concerns

CHAPTER 10

Hair Loss
from Chemotherapy and
Radiation

FIVE HUNDRED SOCIAL WORKERS, NURSES, AND OTHER HEALTH professionals as well as members of the general public are crowded into an auditorium in New York City, where the Chemotherapy Foundation, Inc., and The Mount Sinai School of Medicine are presenting an educational program entitled "Understanding Chemotherapy and the Cancer Experience." They are stunned and puzzled when Ellyn Bushkin, R.N., an assistant director of nursing at the Mount Sinai School of Medicine, and for more than ten years a clinical oncology nurse specialist says, "Of all the side effects from chemo-therapy, alopecia (hair loss) is the most life-threatening one."

Then she continues. "More people refuse chemotherapy because they dread losing their hair, than refuse it for any other reason. And that," she emphasizes, "is life-threatening to the cancer patient."

Her experiences with patients are repeated hundreds of times a day by doctors, nurses and social workers who note that when a person is told they need chemotherapy, the first question they ask is, "Will I lose my hair?"

Hair loss has a profound effect on many people, as we know from the many ways that have been devised to put hair back on heads. But hair loss to the cancer patient has still different meanings. It is, more than anything else in his or her treatment, a visible sign of the illness that tells everyone, "I am getting treatment for cancer."

How Chemotherapy Works

Chemotherapy, which works to destroy cancer cells in all areas of the body, interferes with normal cell growth as well as cancer cell growth. Cells that tend to divide and multiply rapidly, like those in hair follicles, are more vulnerable to this interference than others. The follicles are not destroyed, but the growth cycle is disrupted. And so hair falls out, thins, or ceases to grow. Fortunately, the hair loss is only temporary. Regrowth will often occur even before a person has completed chemotherapy.

Hair loss from chemotherapy is neither inevitable nor predictable. Some chemotherapy drugs affect hair follicles more than others, and some people are not affected as greatly as others. The loss usually follows treatment by two to three weeks. In one scenario the hair falls out at a greater rate than usual and fails to grow back, resulting in a gradual thinning. Or the hair may come out in great clumps in a period of a few days.

There is no correlation between hair loss and the success of the treatment. It is possible that your health is improving even if you don't lose your hair. Conversely, you may be losing your hair although the drugs are not producing the desired positive effects.

Almost all cancer chemotherapy drugs have the potential for hair loss—but some cause it more than others. You should ask your doctor, or the chemotherapy nurse, if hair loss is an expected side effect when you begin chemotherapy.

If You Are Getting Radiation

Radiation therapy is the use of high-energy radiation in the treatment of disease, including cancer. All cells that are exposed to radiation are affected, but normal, healthy cells

recover more quickly than diseased cells. Unlike chemotherapy, radiation does not have a systemic effect. It only
affects those specifically defined areas where it is directed.

Thus, if the radiation is directed where there are hair growing follicles, the hair will fall out and fail to grow for a certain
period of time. As with chemotherapy, people respond differently. This is due, in part, to the dosage, and sometimes,
to the age of the patient.

Extent of Hair Loss

When people think about hair loss they usually think of scalp
hair. Surely this is the part that is most noticeable. However,
hair loss in other areas of the body also occurs. For instance,
the hair follicles of the beard, mustache, eyebrows, eyelashes,
armpits, pubic area and legs and chest can all be affected by
chemotherapy, as can any area that is in the direct path of
the radiation.

Regrowth of Hair

People are usually reassured to learn that hair will grow back.
However, some people are on chemotherapy for several years,
with hair continually falling out and growing back. Sometimes it has just begun to grow back when it falls out again.
This is due to the cyclic nature of the way the drugs are
scheduled, and the natural cycles of hair growth.

In addition to the hair loss, the scalp may become irritated
or flaky. Some people say that using a milder shampoo, and
rubbing olive oil or baby oil into the scalp is helpful.

When hair grows back following chemotherapy—and most
oncologists (physicians who specialize in treating cancer patients) say it always grows back—it tends to grow in softer,
fuller and sometimes in a more youthful color. People sometimes describe it as something like thick vellus hair.

Hair growth does not *always* take place after radiation. If
a strong dosage has been directed towards a cancer that is

lying under the hair follicles, the follicles may be completely destroyed. Then there will be no regrowth.

Preventing Hair Loss

You may have heard that some people use a tourniquet around the scalp while they are receiving an intravenous drip or injection of chemotherapy into their arm. The tourniquet is left on the scalp for about fifteen minutes after the dose is completed, with the intention of protecting the hair follicles in the scalp from the effects of the drug.

Other patients report using a scalp-cooling technique, which makes use of an ice-pack consisting of gel packs molded together with waterproof tape to form a sort of ice-wig. The principle behind the technique is that it constricts the blood vessels in the scalp, decreasing the ability of the drug to get through to the scalp and affect the hair follicles.

In England, ice packs were used in studies with patients who were receiving adriamycin, a drug that almost always causes hair loss and is used to treat many cancers, including breast cancer. The ice packs met with some measure of success, preventing or minimizing hair loss in a significant number of patients. A kind of double-layered rubber bathing cap into which a frozen gel is injected is now being manufactured and distributed commercially. The caps are supposed to be left on the patient for about a half hour before and after treatment.

So why doesn't every oncologist and clinic use one of these methods to prevent hair loss?

They have a good reason. Just as the tourniquet or ice-pack keeps the drug from reaching the scalp and the hair follicles, some feel it could possibly keep the drug from going to the brain. The rationale for the use of chemotherapy is that it is a systemic drug, and has the potential to destroy any cancer cells that may have strayed far (including the brain) from the original tumor.

Ms. Bushkin, who is now a clinical nurse specialist in a large private clinic in a suburb of New York, says, "Anyone who has ever seen cancer spread to the brain in someone getting chemotherapy—but used one of those tourniquets or ice packs—would never want a patient to use one again."

In addition, oncology nurses and physicians say that some people experience extreme dizziness during the period in which they are wearing the ice pack.

Michael A. Goldsmith, M.D., assistant clinical professor of Medicine and Neoplastic Diseases at the Mount Sinai School of Medicine in New York says that tourniquets and ice packs don't always work, and can cause patchy alopecia. He is concerned that the scalp (and maybe even the brain) can become a sanctuary for cancer cells.

Even doctors who believe ice packs pose little danger of cancer spreading to the brain, question their use for other reasons.

Ezra M. Greenspan, M.D., has been in the forefront of chemotherapy treatment for forty years. He is a clinical professor of Medicine (oncology) at the Mount Sinai School of Medicine, the medical director of the Chemotherapy Foundation, and past president of the New York Cancer Society. He says that there is little evidence that the ice packs prevent chemotherapy from going to the brain. "Instead," he says, "you are only keeping the drugs from reaching the scalp, and scalp metastasis (spread) is very rare."

"But," he continues, "the ice packs are not very effective. When a single drug is taken, it may be possible to block it from going to the scalp. But today we use a combination of drugs, given in sequence with intricate timing mechanisms. Many drugs that cause hair loss are taken by mouth, and in those instances there is no way to prevent the hair loss."

If you want to try one of these methods your doctor may allow you to, but some doctors will ask you to sign a release stating that it is your idea, and that you are aware of the possible consequences.

According to most of the health professionals who treat cancer patients, there is really no way to prevent hair loss during chemotherapy. And everyone agrees that hair loss is traumatic. You cannot minimize the effect it has on the emotional well-being of a person to whom it has occurred.

Symbol of Illness

The loss of hair during cancer treatment is, as one patient said, "a double whammy." The hair loss is a concrete symbol, serving notice to everyone that you have cancer. And, at a time when you may not *feel* like yourself, you don't even *look* like yourself.

Arlene Berger, M.S.W., a social worker at Mount Sinai School of Medicine, works with patients who have undergone radiotherapy and chemotherapy. She says that patients often talk about the shock associated with the loss. According to her, "They know they are going to lose their hair, but somehow they're not prepared to find that sometimes it comes out in big clumps, and that it seems to happen almost overnight."

One of the first things women often do when they are recovering from a mild illness is wash their hair, or go to the beauty parlor. They will say, "It's good for my morale, and makes me feel like myself again." Men may look forward to shaving, using their favorite after-shave lotion, and going to their barber for a haircut.

The cancer patient who is undergoing chemotherapy can't make ready use of some of these morale-builders. If hair is falling out, or a beard is failing to grow, these women and men are deprived of their usual ways of raising their spirits.

Hair loss in connection with a serious illness is particularly devastating, according to Jimmie Holland, M.D., Chief of Psychiatric Services at Memorial Sloan-Kettering Cancer Center in New York, because the alteration of a person's appearance can severely affect his or her interactions with others. "Anything," she says, "that makes people look at you differently, has implications that stigmatize you. For example, most people today know that hair loss is related to chemotherapy for cancer so patients are aware that people know something about them that they might not have wanted them to know."

Hair is actually a body part, so Dr. Holland says, "The issues of hair loss are not much different than losing any part of the body in which you have an emotional investment, and that has to do with your sexual attractiveness.

"Most people are affected by hair loss, but it may be especially devastating to those who see themselves primarily in terms of their appearance."

But even those people who have never invested heavily in their looks are very troubled by hair loss. Phyllis Mervis, M.S.W., clinical instructor in Community Medicine (social work) at the Mount Sinai School of Medicine in New York, has worked with cancer patients for more than fifteen years. She says that hair loss becomes a concrete symbol of a powerful illness that can leave you helpless and stripped of dignity. Without hair, people feel undefined, almost like a fetus.

Even when the prognosis is excellent, and a person has good reason to feel that he or she will make a full recovery from this disease, the hair loss may still have a big impact. Carolyn Messner, M.S.W., counsels patients and supervises other social workers at Cancer Care, Inc., a nonprofit social service agency in the greater New York area that helps patients and their families cope with cancer. She explains that people have different perceptions of their hair, but that most people feel it is special. "Sometimes they don't realize that they will lose body hair as well as scalp hair, and this can be just as devastating. Men who lose their beard and body hair, and women who lose their pubic hair, often feel asexual.

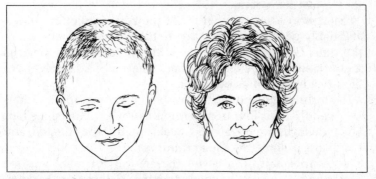

Receiving Chemotherapy
Hair loss from chemotherapy may be patchy or total. A natural-looking wig can make a person feel better as well as look better.

And this loss of self-image comes at a time when they are already vulnerable because of the illness."

Cancer is bad enough. Treatment is not easy. Hair loss seems to add insult to injury.

But there is something you can do about it.

Doing Something About Hair Loss

Many women decide to wear turbans or some other hair covering during the period of hair loss, but countless others decide they want a wig. Their options, as described on pages 129–31, are varied. They can purchase a wig before the hair loss begins, or wait until after it has taken place. Most social workers and nurses who work with patients suggest that patients think about a wig before the hair loss begins, because they can approach the purchase more as a fashion accessory than as a medical necessity.

It can be helpful if a woman purchases an inexpensive synthetic wig before she begins treatment so that later when she looks in the mirror and is depressed by the hair loss, she doesn't have to go out and buy one. If her inclination and budget allow her to purchase an expensive custom-made wig, she will still have the less costly one to wear until it is ready. And many women who *can* afford an expensive wig say they prefer their synthetic one because it makes them feel the hair loss is just temporary.

Men who learn they will lose their hair are often understandably upset. Some just figure they'll wear a hat most of the time. Others decide to "go with it," saying that since so many men have pattern baldness, they will have plenty of bald-headed buddies out there.

Unfortunately, the hair loss from chemotherapy is different than the hair loss from pattern baldness. The fringe hair and sideburns are not spared, eyebrows may be effected, and the beard is sometimes also diminished.

A simple hairpiece is not the answer for men who are suffering hair loss from chemotherapy. If they want to cover their head with hair, they will need a wig. And, as we discussed in chapter 8, wigs for men are expensive.

Custom-Made Wigs for Men

A wig with sideburns will look unnatural if it is not very well made. And that usually means custom made—and expensive. Wigs for men tend to cost upward from $1,400, although many custom designers say that under special circumstances they will adjust their fees for cancer patients.

Harvey Russo of Top Priority makes wigs for many men who are having chemotherapy or have another medical cause of hair loss. Russo says that unless the sideburns are put on a single piece of transparent lace the wig will not look natural. He has noticed that people who are undergoing chemotherapy tend to look sallow, and he adjusts the hair color to compensate for this.

Russo, Jerry Roman of House of Feder and Charles Alfieri all say that if hair loss is expected, men should come in to see them before it occurs. They can make the pattern, begin to create the foundation, and complete the fitting after the hair is lost. This speeds up the delivery of the wig, so that a man can begin to feel like himself sooner. If he has already lost his hair, they ask him to bring a photograph of himself, so that they can create a wig that looks like his own hair.

All three of these men say that when the hair loss is the sudden result of medical or surgical treatment the wig becomes an automatic rush order. If necessary, they will keep someone working overtime to get it finished. Each said, in slightly different words, "You can't imagine what it is like for a man to feel he can't face the world without hair, and how relieved he is when we send him out of here with hair. It is among the most gratifying parts of our work."

Ready-Made Wigs for Men

"Ready-made wigs for men can look satisfactory," says Edith Imre, an internationally recognized hair designer for many, many years. She has seen so many men and women devastated by the loss of hair that she decided to form a nonprofit, charitable organization called the Institute for Loss of Hair. Through the institute, countless wigs are donated to men and women who cannot afford them. Referrals come from doctors, nurses and social workers, or through the American Cancer Society. Edith Imre says, "I have seen people withdraw from all social activity because they couldn't afford to buy a wig. When they go out of here with one of our wigs they gain a renewed interest in life."

She feels that a man's ready-made wig can look very good, *if* it is cut and styled individually. "Unfortunately, most barbers don't really know how to cut a wig, so it may be hard to find someone who can do it properly."

Universal Winners sells wigs for chemotherapy patients as well as hairpieces for men with pattern baldness. Their wigs are not as natural looking as those made by custom designers like Russo, Alfieri and Roman but they are acceptable, and for the man whose need is temporary or who cannot afford a more expensive one, these wigs may be quite satisfactory.

People without hair sometimes complain that ready-made wigs itch, or in other ways irritate the scalp. Harvey Russo, of Top Priority, suggests that people line these wigs with silk. "A wigmaker, or even a handy home sewer, might be able to add this little bit of comfort to an 'itchy' wig," he says.

Permanent Hair Loss

Hair loss may be permanent if high doses of radiation are targeted to a portion of the scalp. In that case, any number of the ways of putting hair back can be employed. However, before embarking on any of the surgical processes, you should discuss it with your cancer specialist.

Hair Loss in Children

Children are also treated for cancer with chemotherapy and radiation, and they too lose their hair. Their reactions to hair loss vary depending on many factors, including age. Many children do not like to wear wigs, and yet they feel vulnerable and exposed without hair, especially if they are teased by schoolmates.

Excellent ready-made and custom-made wigs are available for children, and Edith Imre says the Institute for Loss of Hair has supplied many. It is especially important that children's wigs be natural looking, because other children may tease them if it isn't.

Some professionals who work with children feel that, with counseling, many can be comfortable with their hair loss and feel no need to conceal it except with a hat or scarf.

Costs of Wigs

Women's wigs are available from under $50 for attractive synthetic ones, to a few thousand dollars for custom-made natural hair wigs. Men's wigs are more likely to be expensive: even the synthetic ready-to-wear ones usually cost a few hundred dollars. Custom-made natural wigs are, as we said, considerably more expensive.

The social work department of your local hospital, chapters of American Cancer Society, and other social work agencies may be able to recommend a way that you can get a wig at little or no cost, if you cannot afford to purchase one.

Medical insurance will often pay toward a wig for someone whose hair loss is medical. The cost of the wigs can also be a medical tax deduction.

Ask your physician to write a letter for you, something like this one which Dr. Greenspan does for his patients.

> This patient is under my care for [name of disease] and consequently is receiving chemotherapy. As a result of chemotherapy, the patient suffers from alopecia.
>
> Therefore, it is medically as well as psychologically necessary that [your name] use a prosthesis [wig].

CHAPTER 11

Emotional Aspects
of Hair Loss

My friends at college were all growing their hair long. It seemed that in the 1960s it was the way we announced our philosophical and political beliefs to the world. I envied them having enough hair to "make a statement," because there I was, only a freshman in college and I was losing my hair. I was sure my lack of hair made me an undesirable date, and I spent more time checking my hairline than I did trying to hone my social skills so nobody would care.

Chuck is now a thirty-eight-year-old stockbroker and he can tell the story with a slight smile, but the pain comes through as he recalls those college days. He's come to terms with his loss now, perhaps because his wife likes him just the way he is. But his college graduation gift from his parents was a hair extension, which he abandoned a few years ago when he decided he didn't want to make the time commitment any more.

Don's hair loss started while he was in high school, and his friends teased him about it. Rather than mope around, Don decided to "join in" the jokes, and he would laugh and even refer to himself as a skin-head, a name that soon stuck. But Don didn't really think it was funny, and at home he would spend hours thumbing through magazines looking for ads that promised a cure for baldness. His father had a full head of hair, but his mother's father had been bald at a young age, or so they told him. It wasn't at all consoling, and Don's personality actually changed. He went from being a good, serious student to becoming the class clown—skipping the junior prom (this was in the fifties when they still had proms) and refusing to go away to college for fear of having to meet a lot of new people.

His parents were concerned, and they steered him into seeing a baldheaded therapist. After five sessions, the therapist suggested that maybe Don's problems weren't so deep-rooted after all, and that he ought to try wearing a hairpiece.

I would like to say there was an overnight change in Don's personality, but there wasn't. However, he began to feel that he could now make a good first impression, and that as people got to know him they would forget about his appearance. The hairpiece made it easier to meet new people, but he couldn't wear it for sports or swimming, and he felt it had limited use. In the 1950s little else was available. Eventually, Don had a transplant, and now, still not at ease with sparse hair, he combines it with a hairpiece.

Don's baldness has been a problem to him all of his life, and although he functions well in his professional and personal life—he has a successful career writing special material for comedians, and is married with two daughters— he still tends to hang back when it comes to meeting new people. Indeed, his choice of career reflects his unwillingness to expose himself to the public. But it has been a successful way to channel his class-clown behavior.

Young men who begin to lose their hair in late adolescence suffer tremendously, because it is a time when peer conformity is at its peak. Kids don't realize how painful the hair loss is to him, and jokes they think are harmless can be quite destructive to his still-developing ego. But, even if people don't comment, his mirror tells him the truth, and he has a difficult time adjusting to it.

Men whose hair loss occurred at the start of their careers say that their baldness was a deterrent to getting jobs. Baldness may not be as important in the eye of the beholder as it is in the eye of the beholden, but if a young man feels he lacks an edge because of his hair loss, he will· be self-conscious at the interview, and *that* will work against him. And many men say that they stayed in jobs they didn't like, for fear of going out on interviews. Others say they don't think they are self-conscious about their baldness, but that when they are faced with new situations they suddenly became very aware of their appearance. One young man said he always felt he was missing out on a part of life. When questioned further, he was unable to specify what he was missing, but was convinced that many opportunities—social and business—had been denied him because he was bald.

A young medical student, whom we shall call Jack, said that when he began to lose his hair in his twenties he was struck by the fact that this was the first time in his life that he had no control over something. He had been one of those golden boys who was handsome, a good athlete, a fine student, popular with girls and always knew he could do and be anything he wanted. Indeed, he went from an Ivy League college to a fine medical school, on the way acquiring an attractive young law student as his wife. All was going well in his life. He maintained control over everything: he ate well, worked out regularly and both he and his wife were headed for good careers. In the meantime, their parents were helping to support them, so they didn't even have financial worries.

And then, the hair loss. For Jack, this had many implications. Here was something he couldn't control, and it presented a threat to his self-image.

He began to feel as if he no longer had it all.

Fortunately, he was able to enter one of the Upjohn minoxidil studies, which returned his sense of control to him. His hair loss has stabilized, and it seems to be growing back on the crown.

Lou is an art director at a major advertising agency in New York. A leader in the gay rights movement, he always considered himself a well-adjusted, mature man who didn't place undue importance on esthetics—except, of course in his work.

When he began to lose his hair, he refused, unlike so many others, to see it as a threat to his youth. Instead, he looked at the mirror with his critical artistic eye, and decided he just didn't look right. His face needed a better frame, he said, so he explored the various possibilities of hair replacement.

While Lou's reaction to hair loss seemed more cerebral than psychological, it really was an emotional reaction, which he dealt with in his characteristic, methodically artistic way. And indeed, Lou looked great in the hair extension he finally decided upon.

Ginger's light brown hair was never her crowning glory, she would say, but it served her well. She was a pretty young girl, and an equally attractive woman. But just around the time her son became engaged, Ginger noticed her hair was thinning. By the time the wedding invitations went out, Ginger realized it was more than thinning—she was actually balding at the crown. She thought it was nerves, but her doctor shook his head and said, "I wish it were, because we could do something about it. But it seems to be just common pattern baldness, not so uncommon in women who are menopausal and who are genetically predisposed to hair loss."

Nerves didn't cause her hair loss, but it was soon apparent that the hair loss was doing something terrible to Ginger's nerves. At a time that should have been wonderfully happy, Ginger had a great deal of trouble mustering up the courage to walk down the aisle. The day was saved for her by a clever bridal shop manager who suggested a lovely little hat to match her dress. Eventually, Ginger decided on a wig for special occasions, and she took to wearing hats a lot. As she said, "I'm coping, but I'm not happy about it."

Harry, a thirty-four-year-old history teacher at a local high school, is married to Lisa (not their real names), a computer programmer. They and their three young children live in a lovely house with a spacious backyard and seem to have everything a young couple would want.

But if you say this to Harry, he responds by saying, "Everything? Sure, everything but my hair."

Harry began losing his hair in his mid-twenties, and says his baldness makes him look older, less attractive, and that his students kid him about it. He is sure headwaiters give him that table in the rear because he doesn't enhance the image of the restaurant. And he has already started worrying that his children will be embarrassed to have a baldheaded father. He admits he worries about each hair, and his wife is puzzled at what she terms "his obsession with hair—or his lack of it."

He tried mail-order remedies, but none of them worked. He considered transplants, hair extensions, and hairpieces but has rejected all of them for one reason or another. Lisa says, "It almost seems as if Harry gains some sort of psychic satisfaction from bemoaning his fate."

Harry is mourning his lost hair, is unable to come to terms with the loss or do something about replacing it. But is the intensity of his reaction a manifestation of other unresolved problems in his life, with which he would prefer not to deal? Focusing on the hair loss prevents him from having to do so.

This is not to say that people who are upset about hair loss, who feel insecure and self-conscious about it, are necessarily suffering from an emotional disorder. No, indeed. We all need that extra edge, and looking good is an extra edge.

Many of today's therapists recognize that changing one area of your life—appearance, for instance—can change how you and others perceive you, and can ultimately change your feelings about yourself as a person.

What about Harry? Would a hair replacement solve his problems?

It would solve his hair problem, but he would then have to face whatever else was bothering him. Harry has been, as they say in the jargon of mental health practitioners, defending against his anxieties and feelings of inadequacy by displacing everything that goes wrong in life on his lack of hair. By rejecting all possible ways of replacing his hair, he will never find out if his students would treat him with more respect, if headwaiters would give him a better table, and if his children would like him better if he had hair.

Although some people may disagree, I feel that Harry really

should try a hair replacement. It would give him a chance to recognize that he has problems, and then do something about them. And who knows, maybe hair would just make him feel better about himself.

Most people are not as uptight as Harry about their hair loss. They are unhappy, and self-conscious about it, and often bemoan their fate. But they accept it, or seek a way to grow it back or put it back. They may look with envy at men old enough to be their fathers who still have a full head of hair, but they have friends, lovers and wives, and they hold all kinds of jobs. They may spend considerably more time and money on their hair than men who haven't lost their hair, but they don't allow their hair, or lack of it, to be the central focus of their lives.

SECTION SIX

Making the Most of
What You Have

CHAPTER 12

Caring for Your Hair

WHETHER YOU STILL HAVE A GOOD DEAL OF HAIR THAT IS THIN-
ning or receding, or just a nice thick one-inch horseshoe
fringe, that remaining hair is entitled to the most tender loving care you can give it.

According to Vera Price, M.D., associate clinical professor
of Dermatology of the University of California, San Francisco,
the key rule of good hair care is to handle it as gently as you
can. She suggests that to minimize wear and tear you use a
bone or plastic comb with round tipped separated bristles.

Albert Lefkovits, M.D., assistant clinical professor of Dermatology at the Mount Sinai School of Medicine, New York,
adds, "Be wary of heavy brushing because it will lead to
physical trauma and then to breakage. If your hair is at all
damaged, use a soft brush, or gently groom with a comb
instead of a brush."

Shampooing Your Hair

Thorough shampooing of your hair is the first line of defense
against hair and scalp problems: *how* you wash your hair is
just as important as *what* you use.

"Shampoo the hair gently with the fingertips, not the fin-
gernails," Dr. Price says. Hair can be washed daily, *if* you

don't use too harsh a shampoo. If the scalp or hair is very oily it probably needs daily shampoo.

Types of Shampoos

It has been a long time since people used a bit of their favorite soap to wash their hair. Soap can leave a dull, sticky film on the hair, one which is difficult to remove even with repeated rinsing. Today's shampoos are composed of synthetic detergents, which wash and rinse well even in hard water, getting rid of all that soapy residue.

Synthetic shampoos are formulated for oily, normal, and dry hair. A quick study of the labels will tell you if they are suitable for your kind of hair and for the frequency with which you want to wash it. Most experts seem to feel that if you wash your hair every day you are probably wiser to use a gentle or normal shampoo. A shampoo that is formulated for oily hair may be too harsh for daily use, and can even remove too much of the hair's natural sebum, making it dull and difficult to manage. Harsh chemicals can also damage the hair cuticle. This will expose the cortex to the environmental effects of sun, wind, chemicals and dirt, and cause hair breakage.

Shampoos are often described as being low pH, or pH balanced, or nonalkaline. What does this mean?

A scale which represents the relative acidity (or alkalinity) of a solution is described as pH. A scale of 7.0 is neutral, below 7.0 is acid, and above 7.0 is alkaline.

For purposes of cleansing, soap is highly alkaline. Since this is damaging to the hair, acid is added to most shampoos to lower the pH value. The acids, such as citric acid, make hair easier to handle, reducing flyaway hair. Which is why, years ago before shampoos were developed, people often used a lemon rinse following their soapy hair wash.

The Right Shampoo for You

Many dermatologists say that any mild shampoo containing animal protein will give more body to the hair than those with natural protein such as egg or gelatin, and that dry hair will benefit from a shampoo with lanolin, cholesterol, and lecithin emollients, or oily additives.

Several of these experts say that hair may build up some sort of natural tolerance to a particular brand of shampoo, and they suggest that you frequently switch brands. George Roberson, successful New York hair stylist and author of *Men's Hair* (Rawson, 1985), recommends that you keep a few different kinds of shampoo in the shower, and change off regularly, rather than switching every time you use one up.

He also suggests that you use professional products for the hair—the kind they sell in beauty supply stores or through barbers and beauty parlors. The big advertised brands contain a lot of ingredients that dry out the hair, and, he says that often you're paying for their advertising and packaging.

"Don't think your hair should squeak after you finish washing it, because that means you hair is really too dry, and you have probably used a shampoo that stripped all the oil off of it," he warns.

Conditioners, Rinses and Thickeners

Many people today consider a conditioner to be part of their regular shampoo routine, and surely this can minimize tangling and make combing easier. Dr. Vera Price says, "This lessens the force you apply when combing hair and reduces hair damage."

George Roberson likes conditioners and finishing rinses because they seal and tighten the cuticle of the hair, coat the shaft, and make strands thicker so that hair has more shine and the static is removed. "But be careful," he says, "because so-called cream rinses can coat and weigh the hair down."

Some of these conditioners contain body-building proteins, and are acidic, which counteracts excessive pH in your shampoo. Deep-down conditioners which you leave on the hair for five minutes or more can penetrate and coat the hair, and do just what regular conditioners do—only more so.

But conditioners can be a catch-22 for people with thinning hair. They make hair more manageable, but they can also make it look limp. Be careful of heavy cream rinses, and

stay with light protein conditioners. Roberson suggests, "If
you use only a dot, a dime-sized dollop, your hair will get
the benefits without the heaviness."

He also suggests you try one of the thickening agents like
THICKET, made by Madric, Ltd. which contains a wax. He
says it lies on top of hair strands, and a quick combing or
brushing fluffs it up for a natural, thicker look. He more
strongly recommends another type of thickener which contains animal proteins that are absorbed into the hair shafts,
instead of just lying on top of the hair strands. It's called
Mahdeen's MEDI-PRO, and Roberson says you may have to
get it at a beauty supply store.

None of these products really cause the hair to become
thicker, they just make it look that way—until you wash it
out in the next day's shampoo.

After the Shampoo

Dr. Vera Price recommends that you towel-dry your hair by
patting it, rather than vigorously rubbing it. "Wet hair is
weaker and more easily damaged than dry hair," she explains, "so it needs to be combed especially carefully and
minimally."

Fluffing up your hair and then using a hair dryer can
certainly make it look like you have more hair. But Dr. Albert
Lefkovits pleads, "Be careful of high heat on those hair driers.
It only takes a few more minutes to dry your hair with a
lower heat, and it can really avoid damage to your hair."

Hair Dressings and/or Sprays

Remember the "greasy kid stuff," otherwise known as hair
pomades? They have been pretty well supplanted by hair
sprays in pump dispensers (better than aerosol cans) and
setting lotions, at least for the man or woman whose hair is
thinning. If you still prefer a "dressing" type of product, try
a water-based gel rather than an oil-based one, which will
flatten the hair and tend to slick it down.

Special Problems

Hair and scalp itchy and flaky? Check the humidity in your bedroom at night—if low, it can cause your skin and hair (as well as your throat and nasal passages) to feel very dry. Get a humidifier for the room, and shampoo your hair less often, using a formula specially designed for dry hair.

Is your hair oily only hours after you washed it? Bet you also have ring around the collar. Oily complexion and hot humid weather go together with oily hair. Shampoo daily, and alternate your regular shampoo with one specifically formulated for oily hair.

Fine white scales flaking off your scalp onto your new blue blazer, or best new cashmere sweater? It might be dandruff, although sometimes just lack of frequent washing can produce the same effect. Simple dandruff is often controlled by frequent washing, occasionally using some of the anti-dandruff shampoos sold at drug stores. If dandruff persists, see a dermatologist.

Basic Care

Basic hair and scalp care begins with good, frequent shampooing, and gentle handling of hair. Conditioners, rinses and thickeners can make hair look and feel better—temporarily—but they will not really change the structure of the hair, and will need to be repeated at regular intervals.

If you value your hair:
• Avoid traction and friction.
• Avoid chemical damage from permanents, dyes and bleaches.
• Avoid too much sun.

Treating your hair with tender loving care, and using the right products can work wonders. As can the proper styling and color, which we will discuss in the next chapter.

CHAPTER 13

A Little Honest Deception: Styling and Color

ALTHOUGH YOU'VE TRIED EVERYTHING TO KEEP YOUR HAIR, IT'S going, going, but not quite gone. You're not yet ready to think about a way of putting it back, or perhaps you're a middle-aged man or woman who has decided that your hair loss is fairly stabilized, and you just want to *look* like you have more hair.

"Please, please," all our experts say, "don't part it down near the ear and swing it across your forehead. If you think that makes you look like you have a lot of hair, you're only fooling yourself."

Haircuts and Placement of Part

Listen to Ray Olsen, top-notch stylist at one of Act II Haircutters' dozen salons in New York and New Jersey. He cuts men's and women's hair, and he says, "If you try to camouflage hair loss too much you just make it more obvious. Don't try to hide the loss, but instead have your hair cut shorter and closer to the scalp."

He also warns against teasing hair, because it looks unnatural, can harm the hair, and will actually make the scalp show more.

George Roberson echoes Olsen on the strand of hair plastered across the head. He says, "If the part is below the ear everyone knows there's a bald spot below that long strand, even if they can't see it. It doesn't make you look younger, but something like an old troll holding onto the last dying hair strand. And plastered hair feels stiff as a rock, so you can't dare let anyone touch it."

He says that your hair can look thicker if you avoid any definite part, and he encourages men to groom their hair with their hands, which can give it direction and lift. "Avoid combing and brushing which exerts pressure and flattens the hair. When you come out of the shower just comb your hair with your fingers. If you leave hair a little wild, it can camouflage a receding hairline," he tells his clients.

David Crespin, an attractive, balding Manhattan hair stylist, cuts men's and women's hair to fit their looks and lifestyle. He keeps his own three-inch horseshoe fringe short, but full, and warns against letting it grow too thick, as if to make up for the lost hair. "You'll look like you have earmuffs," he says, "and it will just call more attention to your bald area."

A slight moving of the part to give the illusion of more hair is fine, says Crespin, but some men carry it too far and end up with that look that makes other people worry everytime the wind blows.

Francisco, a hair stylist with Vidal Sassoon, has a whole bag of tricks he uses on men with thinning or balding hair. "A little cheating on the part is all right," he says, "but you must look at the shape of the head as well as the hair. For instance, if a man has a wide head, moving the part too far to one side will accentuate that wideness, and so even though he may look like he has more hair, it will not be a flattering style for him. Ordinarily, he would look better with his part near the center.

"Men's foreheads usually do not recede symmetrically, so unless that pattern of hair growth prohibits it, if you move the part away from the most receding side you will reduce the bald look. If the bald spot is in the back I suggest cutting surrounding hair closer to the scalp than the rest of the hair, so the bald spot doesn't look like a sand trap," Francisco says.

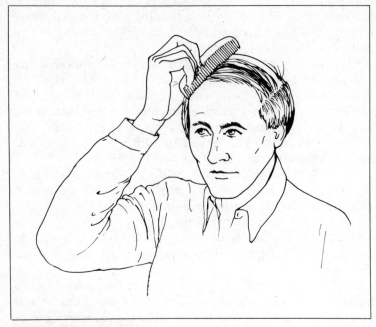

Too Much Deception
Trying to hide baldness by moving the part all the way to the ear doesn't really fool people.

No More Long Hair ... Please

Our experts all agreed that the same guy or gal who looked fine with long hair in the 1960s will now look ridiculous in that now if he or she has begun to thin or bald. Usually hair thins at the same time as it balds, and long hair will look stringy and unkempt. Men in particular begin to look as if they haven't been to the barber since they bought those first sandals and beads.

"Shorter hair stands up better because it automatically has more resilience and lift. It's bouncier because weighted length doesn't pull it down," says Charles Hix in his best seller, *Looking Good: A Guide for Men* (Hawthorne Books, Inc., 1977; Wallaby, 1978).

The best way to avoid calling attention to your problem

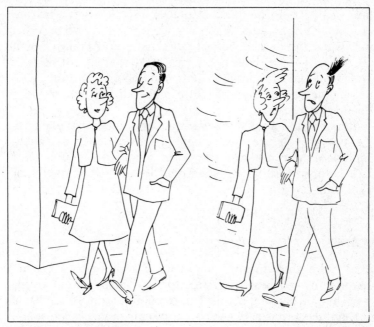

Stay Out of the Wind
The man with plastered-down hair is in trouble if the wind blows in the wrong direction.

is to keep hair in proportion to itself and to your facial features. In women, soft bangs can cover a receding forehead. But long hair will not look youthful, or deflect the eye from a balding area. Instead it will serve to highlight it.

Body Waves and Permanents

"Wavy and curly hair looks thicker and fuller, so if you are not blessed with it naturally, consider having a permanent," says Ray Olsen.

Francisco also likes a body wave, and says that if the hair can support side fullness, it will give a thicker look. "But be careful of that dog's ear look with too much and too curly hair on the sides, if there isn't much on top," he advises.

Roberson recommends body waves because they can chemically alter the hair's structure, giving it more texture and body. "Sometimes," he says, "you can have your stylist just wave the hair on top of your head, and then blend it more easily with the bulkier hair on the sides and back. If your problem is general, rather than specific thinning, you could have a full body wave to make all the hair on your head look thicker."

Remember our previous warnings about the risks of chemical damage: be sure a permanent is done carefully in a good, reputable salon, and don't do it the same day as you do your hair color or just before you are off for a week of surfing or swimming.

Color

Hair color that doesn't stand out is another trick recommended by our experts. Francisco recommends highlighting dark hair, especially if your complexion if light. He says that when the contrast between hair and scalp or face is too sharp, the bald look is accentuated.

George Roberson likes a good professional color rinse made up of equal parts shampoo, twenty-volume peroxide and hair color applied to damp hair. "Color rinses don't necessarily change the color of hair, but they add body and lots of shine, which is just the right prescription for thinning hair.

"After your twenties, hair just isn't shiny anymore, so most men as well as women need a little color to make the hair shiny and luscious. The color can even make hair thicker and coarser looking."

Dermatologists warn against too-harsh dyes that may damage hair (albeit temporarily) or cause an allergic reaction. So be sure you have it done by a reputable and responsible salon, or use a good brand-name home product. If you have any history of allergies, do a small patch test to make sure you're not hypersensitive to the hair color. Using an absorbent cotton-dipped applicator, apply a small amount of the coloring solution in the bend of your elbow or behind either ear where your hairline begins. Leave the test spot untouched for twenty-four hours, and if there is any abnormal reaction such as burning, itching, swelling, skin abrasions, eruption, or irritation around the test area, don't use the product. Wait a few days and then try a patch test using another brand.

Diverting the Eye

There's nothing wrong with a little honest deception, if it can draw attention to your face instead of your head. "A stunning beard will make eyes focus on the beard rather than hair," says George Roberson, but he advises people to be sure the beard suits the face. A long beard on a long face can make the face look even longer, and call attention to the top of the head.

Ray Olsen likes beards or mustaches because it makes men feel as if they can still grow hair, and gives them something to fuss over. "Watch proportion," he and all our experts say. "Be patient, beards and mustaches don't grow overnight."

Charles Hix says growing them isn't too complicated. First, you stop shaving the areas in which you want growth, allowing up to six weeks before a mustache or beard is dense enough to do any real styling.

"A beard doesn't hide a good face. It can accent one when kept in proportion with the hair on the head, forming a continuation of the hairstyle. Thus, short, neat hair atop demands the symmetry of neat, short hair below," he says in *Looking Good.*

Our experts agree that the thinning or balding head calls for short, neat hair atop, so please *don't* overdo the beard. Remember, just a little deception is all we really want.

A Little Compensation

Your hair is thinning or balding, it isn't growing back, and it's too soon to put it back, so you're just going to stand in front of that mirror every day counting hairs on the top of your head. Right? Wrong, I hope.

Change what you can, and learn to live with (if not accept)

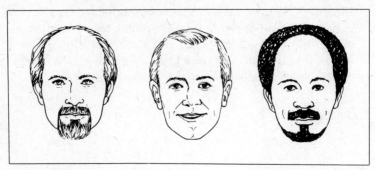

Looking Good
A neat, short haircut, a mustache or a beard helps divert the eye
from hair loss.

what you can't. Make that hair look fuller, if you can, and if
you can't, do something about the rest of you.

Get that body back into shape. Join a gym, and lose those
extra few pounds. You do have control over those things.

Take a course, make some new friends, do some volunteer
work, and *stop* looking in every mirror.

You notice your hair more than anyone else does.

Afterword

MY SON'S FRIEND TOM ASKED TO READ THE MANUSCRIPT DIrectly from my word processor so he could get a head start on the answer to his galloping hair loss.

My old friend Liz doesn't dwell on her thinning hair, but prefaces every phone call with, "How's the book coming? Anything new for me?" And then tells me about her new stylist who has done wonders.

Twenty-eight-year-old Marc said, "I'll be happy to read your book, Mary-Ellen, but you'll just have to excuse me if I decide to grow bald gracefully."

For all the Marcs in the world, there are millions of men and women who, to paraphrase Dylan Thomas, burn and rage, refusing to bald gentle through this good life. For them, this book was written.

You can now deal with your hair loss in your own way. The decision is yours. You know how hair grows, and what can cause its loss. You have the wisdom to know when you *can't* stop the hair loss, but you also now know about hair regrowth, hair replacement, and professional tricks to make your remaining hair look better. You have learned about the wondrous new drug, minoxidil, that is growing hair on heads all over the country. You have learned about the surgical and cosmetic improvements and developments that can put hair on everyone's head, including yours.

But please, before you rush ahead and decide on any of

the methods described here, check out the professional qualifications of any medical or cosmetic practitioners you are
considering. Your county medical society can usually give
you names of physicians in your area who are trained to do
the procedures which you want to consider. You can check
qualifications of any physician in the Directory of Medical
specialists at your local library. Before you do anything, check
with your family doctor.

Contact the Better Business Bureau in your area to see if
any complaints have been lodged against any clinic or salon
before you let them touch your scalp or precious remaining
hair.

You *can* reverse hair loss—there is no longer any reason
to bemoan your fate or to try untested products or services
one after another. Your clothes, your home, your car, and
your career, as well as your friends and family, all reflect the
way you feel about yourself. Your hair should do the same.
If you feel you are someone who should have hair—then—
   Go to it!

Glossary

Acidity

Natural state of hair is acidic. Acidity is a term which describes the concentration of hydrogen in a solution. Acidity and its opposite, alkalinity, are measured on a pH scale of 0 to 14. The lower the pH number, the higher the acidity. (See alkalinity; pH.)

Acne

Inflammatory skin eruption, involving sebaceous glands. It is often characterized by pimples on the face.

Aldactone

Trade name for spironolactone, a drug often prescribed for hypertension. It can also arrest hair loss and sometimes cause hair growth.

Alkalinity

The opposite of acidity, representing an absence of hydrogen ions in a solution. A soap or shampoo which is alkaline can remove the delicate cuticle from the hair shaft, causing hair to tangle and be difficult to comb. The higher the pH number, the higher the alkalinity. (See Acidity; pH.)

Alopecia

Partial or complete lack of hair. The term is used for baldness resulting from pattern baldness, congenital conditions, medication, illness, skin disease, trauma and any other causes.

Alopecia areata

A disease, in which the body forms antibodies against some of the hair follicles. It is characterized by small, smooth, round or oval patches of baldness on the scalp or beard, and may clear up spontaneously within a few months, or may persist. Treatment for alopecia areata is often, but not always, successful.

Alopecia totalis

An uncommon condition in which there is no hair on the scalp. It can develop from alopecia areata, or result from some other cause.

Alopecia universalis

An uncommon condition in which there is no hair on any part of the body. It can develop from alopecia areata, or result from another cause.

Amino acids

The essential peptides and proteins required for life, which act as building blocks in the construction and functioning of the human body. An amino acid called cysteine is found in keratin, an important ingredient of hair (See Keratin.)

Anagen

The growing stage in the hair growth cycle is called the anagen phase. About 85 to 90 percent of a person's hair is always in the anagen phase, which lasts from two to five years.

Anagen effluvium

Loss of hair that is supposed to be in the growing, or anagen phase. This frequently follows chemotherapy or radiation.

Analgesic

A drug that can relieve pain without producing anesthesia or loss of consciousness. Mild analgesics include aspirin and Tylenol.

Androgen

A collective term for a group of male sex hormones, found in both men and women.

Androgenic baldness

(See Pattern baldness)

Anterior scalp
Front of the head. A receding forehead may be referred to as anterior hair loss or baldness.

Antibiotics
A drug which can destroy or interfere with the development of infections, bacteria, and other living organisms.

Antibodies
Part of the body's own defense against foreign substances causing, among other things, rejection of organ transplants from other people.

Autograft
A graft taken from one part of a person's body and transplanted to another part. Hair plugs, tunnel grafts, etc., nisms.

Autoimmunity
A condition in which the body reacts unfavorably against its own tissues and substances.

Axillary hair
Underarm hairs which develop during puberty, with the onset of the introduction of sex hormones into the bloodstream.

Bacteria
Single-celled microorganisms which can be, but are not necessarily, harmful.

Beard
Facial hair which develops at puberty in response to circulating male hormones. Men normally develop a beard, but women with an excess of male hormones, or a shortage of female hormones, may also develop facial hair.

Biopsy (verb: to biopsy; noun: a biopsy)
Removal from the body of a small piece of living tissue, which is then examined microscopically to establish or confirm a diagnosis.

Biotin
Sometimes referred to as Vitamin H, biotin is part of the vitamin B complex. Involved in the metabolism of proteins, fats, and carbohydrates.

Castration (surgical and hormonal)

Castration is generally used to describe the surgical removal of men's testicles or women's ovaries, significantly reducing male hormones in men, and female hormones in women. It is an appropriate procedure for certain cancers which are dependent on hormones for their growth. Castration can also be achieved by the administration of hormones. In males, castration before puberty will prevent any significant hair loss, and after puberty can arrest hair loss, but not restore hair that is already lost.

Chemotherapy

Treatment of illness by drugs or medication which can reach all parts of the body. The term is a general one, but is most often used to refer to the treatment of cancer by drugs which can interfere with and destroy cancer cell growth.

Cicatrical alopecia

Baldness caused by scar tissue which has developed from medical or physical assault to the head, infection, chemicals or burns.

Common baldness

(See Pattern baldness.)

Congenital

Present at birth. A congenital condition may or may not be inherited.

Cortex

Cortex usually refers to the outer layer of a body organ or other structure, but in hair it refers to most of the inner structure. The medulla is at the center, and the cuticle forms the outermost layer of the hair. The fibers of the cortex, which are made of keratin protein, separate and cause split ends if damaged.

Cortisone

An anti-inflammatory medication. Cortisones are synthetic forms of steroid hormones which occur naturally in the body. They are used to treat many conditions, among which are alopecia areata.

Cosmetologist

An individual who concentrates on care of the skin.

Qualifications and licensing may vary in different states.
Cuticle
The outer surface of hair, composed of overlapping scales made of translucent, colorless keratin protein. The cuticle gives hair its luster and shine and also provides some of its strength. The cuticle is damaged slightly by alkaline soaps and shampoos. It can be damaged severely by harsh chemicals. Shampoos low in pH, and conditioners can restore the cuticle.
Dandruff
An excessive amount of scaly, flaky material formed on and shed from the scalp. It is often caused by seborrhea, and can be helped by frequent washing, and by occasionally using an antidandruff shampoo.
Dermatologist
A licensed physician who is trained and specializes in diagnosis and medical and surgical treatment of skin disorders. Disorders of the scalp and hair are included in this specialty.
Diabetes
A metabolic condition in which the body has diminished or no ability to produce or use the hormone insulin, which metabolizes carbohydrates such as sugar. Frequently, there is excessive excretion of urine. Hair loss is among the symptoms of increased levels of sugar in the blood.
Dihydroprogesterone (DHP)
A derivative of progesterone. DHP competes with 5 alpha reductcase, reducing the amount available to make DHT and leading to reduction of the rate of alopecia.
Dihydrotestosterone (DHT)
A derivative of the male hormone, testosterone. DHT assumes responsibility in men for the large terminal hairs on the outside of the ears, nostrils, beard, chest, arms and legs, and upper pubic area. It also bonds together with hair in certain "target" follicles, causing miniaturization of the follicles and leading to baldness. A catalyzing enzyme, 5 alpha reductase, transforms or metabolizes testosterone into DHT.

Dinitrochlorobenzene (DNCB)
A strong chemical which is used as a treatment for alopecia areata.

Donor area (and donor plugs)
The area, usually on the back of the scalp, from which skin with hair-bearing follicles is removed for transplanting elsewhere on the scalp.

Double-blind study
A scientific study, often used to study a new drug, in which neither the investigator (person/s conducting study) or subjects (those being studied) know who is getting the drug and who is getting something else.

Edema
An abnormal accumulation of fluid in tissues in some area of the body, which can be caused by a number of factors. Most often, it is perceived by the patient as swelling.

Endocrine system
A network of glands and tissues that secrete hormones directly into the bloodstream. The endocrine system includes the brain, ovaries, testicles, kidneys, adrenals, thyroid gland, pituitary glands, pancreas, and the linings of the stomach and intestines. Secretions from the endocrine glands affect various processes throughout the body, as metabolism and growth. Disorders of the endocrine system are sometimes associated with hair loss.

Enzyme
Proteins in the body which, acting singly or in combination, catalyze chemical reactions in the body. An enzyme, 5 alpha reductase, converts testosterone to DHT, which contributes to baldness.

Estrogen
One of a group of hormones that causes female secondary sex characteristics. Estrogen is formed in the ovaries in women, and in the adrenal glands in both men and women.

5 alpha reductase
A catalyzing enzyme that converts testosterone to dihy-

drotestosterone (DHT), which then miniaturizes the follicles, leading to baldness.

Flaps

(See Hair transplants.)

Follicle

A pouchlike depression in the skin, formed before birth, from which hair grows. Follicles require a normal amount of oxygen, blood supply, nutrients, growth, thyroid hormones and the "right" heredity to produce hair growth.

Friction alopecia

Loss of hair developing from friction. It can be caused by constantly wearing a hat, wig or some other close fitting head covering, or from rubbing the head on a pillow. Hair can break off so close to the scalp that it looks as if it has come out by the roots, but if the friction ceases, hair will almost always grow back.

Fusion

A process by which synthetic or human hair is linked to a person's own hair. Fusion makes use of a water insoluble glue that forms a chemical bond with the hair.

General anesthesia

A type of anesthesia which induces absence of sensation and consciousness. When a person has surgery performed under general anesthesia, there is no pain or recollection of the procedure.

Genes

A biological unit of genetic material within a DNA molecule which is capable of self-replication. Some genes have variable penetrance, which means that a gene won't always produce its effect. That may explain why baldness does not always manifest itself, even when it is likely that the gene is inherited.

Genetic baldness

(See Pattern baldness.)

Glands

Organs in the body that secrete materials onto the surface of the body or into the blood system.

Hairpiece

A partial replacement of hair, usually intended to blend in with a person's own hair. Hairpieces are sometimes referred to as toupees.

Hair shaft

The exposed hair, covered by a cuticle which acts as a protective shield.

Hair transplants (including plugs, strips, flaps, miniplugs)

A surgical procedure in which scalp grafts, including hair-bearing follicles and skin, are removed from one area of the head and transplanted to another. These grafts may be small four millimeter plugs, smaller miniplugs, larger strips, or flaps of skin and hair which are swiveled from one part of the scalp to another.

Hormones

A term generally used to describe chemicals produced by the endocrine glands (but also produced elsewhere), which can initiate, control or regulate the activity of an organ or group of cells in another area of the body. Steroid hormones include sex hormones that affect hair growth and hair loss.

Hypersensitive

An excessive allergic type reaction and response of the immune system to a particular stimulus.

Hypertension

High blood pressure.

Implants

A procedure that was performed during the 1970s. It involved the implanting of synthetic hair directly into the scalp. Serious adverse effects were reported, and the procedure was banned by the FDA in 1983. Not to be confused with suture stitching process or tunnel grafts.

Intravenous

The term is often used to describe an injection or "drip" of fluid directly into a vein.

Keratin

A strong elastic protein, rich in sulphur, found in each strand of hair and in finger and toenails.

Lanugo
A very fine, sometimes colorless hair with which babies are born. Lanugo hair, more often known as vellus hair, is the downy, almost invisible hair that covers most of an adult's body and a bald person's scalp.

Lateral scalp
The sides of the scalp.

Local anesthesia
A substance which reduces or eliminates pain in a limited area of the body.

Lupus
A group of diseases, some of which are systemic and others which only relate to the skin. Hair loss may be associated with lupus.

Male pattern baldness
(See Pattern baldness.)

Matrix
An intercellular substance deep inside the hair follicle.

Medulla
The most internal part of a structure or organ, as in the hair.

Melanins
The pigmenting granules within the keratin fibers of the hair which determine the hair color. Melanin decreases with age, resulting in gray and white hair.

Menopause
The period of cessation of menstruation, sometimes reffered to as "change of life." The female hormones which counteract some of the effects of the androgens are decreased, leading to hair thinning or some baldness.

Metabolic
Basic chemical processes, resulting in growth, generation of energy, elimination of wastes, and other bodily functions. Certain metabolic disorders can cause hair loss.

Miniplugs
(See Hair transplants.)

Minoxidil
An effective prescription drug that lowers blood pressure

by relaxing and enlarging certain small blood vessels so that blood flows through them more easily. Bodily hair growth was noted to be a side effect of the drug. Minoxidil, when applied to the scalp in lotion form, can cause hair growth on the scalp in many people who have balded for a variety of reasons.

Papilla

The small root area at the base of hair. It receives nutrients from the follicle, which are needed for hair growth.

Patch test

A skin test to determine if there is an allergy or other adverse reaction to a substance.

pH

A scale which indicates relative acidity and alkalinity concentrations. A value of 7.0 is neutral, below 7.0 is acid, and above 7.0 is alkaline.

Pigment

Colored material which is produced in the body, as melanin.

Plugs

(See Hair transplants)

Polysorbate

An emulsifier used in the preparation of pharmacologic products. It is an FDA-approved common food additive.

Posterior scalp

The back of the head.

Progesterone

A hormone which, in its natural state, prepares a woman's uterus for the fertilized ovum and maintains pregnancy. It is often prescribed topically or by injection into the scalp, to stop hair loss in men and women.

Propylene glycol

A colorless liquid, used in various solutions, which acts as a solvent. It is often used in combination with pulverized minoxidil tablets to produce a lotion to apply to the scalp.

Proteins

A group of organic compounds, containing amino acids, which are needed for growth and repair of animal tissue.

Puberty

Period of time during which male and female hormones begin to circulate throughout the body, marking the beginning of secondary sexual characteristics and sexual maturity.

Pubic hair

Hair that grows in the groin area, beginning at puberty. Usually darker than scalp hair, it tends to be short and curly.

Pulverize

Pound, crush, or grind to a dust-like substance.

PUVA

A treatment for alopecia areata in which a light sensitizing medication (psoralen) is applied topically or taken internally, followed by exposure to ultraviolet light (UVA).

Radiation

The emission of energy, rays or waves. Radiation therapy is the use of high-energy radiation in the treatment of disease, including cancer.

Recipient area (and recipient plugs)

Area in which a transplant is placed. The donor plugs that are moved from the back of the scalp to the crown or front of the scalp are then called recipient plugs.

Rejection

The body's recognition of a transplant or graft as foreign, resulting in an adverse or negative reaction.

Rheumatoid arthritis

A chronic, sometimes deforming disease that has an auto-immune component.

Root

The lowest part of an organ or structure which is attached to something. The hair root grows out of the follicle.

Scalp

The skin which covers the head, excluding face and ears.

Scalp reduction

A surgical procedure in which portions of the bald scalp are removed, and the ends are pulled together and surgically stitched. Transplant surgery usually follows scalp reduction.

Scalp stretching

A new surgical procedure in which a small incision is made into the scalp, and two silicone inflatable bags are inserted. These bags allow the skin on the scalp to stretch and grow, permitting subsequent scalp reduction that is more extensive than would have been possible before.

Scar tissue

Scar tissue on the scalp results from any type of burn or cut that extends below the outer skin area. It usually destroys the hair follicles, preventing hair growth.

Sebaceous glands

Small, fatty glands, found in the hair follicles throughout the body, which secrete the oily sebum into the hair and surrounding skin.

Seborrhea

A general term for a common skin condition in which there is an overproduction of sebum, resulting in oily skin or hair.

Seborrhea capitis

A condition in which people have a perpetually oily scalp and hair, and excessively thick dandruff scales and crust, soreness and itching. It can lead to hair loss.

Senescent alopecia

Diffuse thinning of hair in men and women in later years.

Sideburns

The growth of hair down the sides of the face in front of the ears, ending at midpoint of the ears.

Squaric acid dibutyl ester

A strong chemical used in treatment of alopecia areata.

Steroids

A closely related group of chemical substances, comprising many hormones, vitamins and other compounds found in the body naturally. Natural and synthetic derivatives of the steroids are also used as treatment for many medical conditions.

Strips

(See Hair transplants.)

Superior scalp

Upper portion of the scalp.

Suture
 The medical term for a stich.
Systemic
 Pertaining to the entire body, rather than just a particular part of it.
Tagamet
 The trade name for cimetidine, a drug commonly prescribed for ulcers, which can also arrest hair loss.
Tinea capitis
 A fungus infection of the hair and scalp, known as ringworm. It is more frequently found in children than adults.
Telogen
 The resting and shedding phase of the hair growth cycle, lasting from two to six months.
Telogen effluvium
 Excessive hair loss during the telogen phase.
Terminal hairs
 The hair which grows on the scalps of children (after babyhood) and adults. After puberty it grows on the faces of males, and in the pubic and axillary areas of men and women.
Testosterone
 A naturally occurring male hormone found in both men and women.
Thyroidism
 A medical disorder of the thyroid gland.
Topical
 To the surface of some part of the body.
Tourniquet
 A wide constricting band usually applied to a part of the body near the site of life-threatening bleeding. However, a tourniquet is sometimes applied to the scalp in an attempt to keep chemotherapy from reaching the scalp and causing hair loss.
Traction alopecia
 A condition in which hair that has been pulled too tightly begins to fall out, and in some instances, doesn't grow back.

Transsexual

A person who has had medical and surgical procedures to alter their sex from male to female, or female to male.

Trichotilomania

A compulsion, usually unconscious, to pull or tear out hair, often resulting in patchy or diffuse alopecia. It is more common in children and the elderly, but occurs in all age groups.

Tunnel graft

A graft of skin which is surgically removed from another part of the body and attached to the head, allowing a hairpiece to be securely anchored to the scalp by means of clips.

Vellus hairs

Downy, almost invisible hair that covers most of an adult's body and sometimes a bald person's scalp. Following hair loss from chemotherapy, the first regrowth is often vellus hair.

Ventilation

The technical term for double-knotting or crocheting individual strands of natural or synthetic hair to a wig or hairpiece.

Vertex

The highest point, or crown, of the head.

Weaving

A procedure by which a person's own hair is braided tightly, and replacement hair is woven into it. Some of the newer weaving methods, which may or may not involve braiding, are called by other names, such as hair extension.

Wigs

A complete replacement for a person's own hair, placed over existing hair, or over a bald head.

Zinc

A mineral that is necessary to human life for growth. A serious zinc deficiency can cause lack of growth in children, and hair loss at any age.

Sources to Consult

The following organizations offer a referral service, and will provide you with the names of three surgeons in your geographical area who are trained in transplant surgery.

American Academy of Dermatology, Inc.
1567 Maple Avenue, Evanston, Illinois 60201
312/869-3954

They also can provide you with names of members of the American Association of Cosmetic Surgeons, and the American Society of Dermatologic Surgery.

American Academy of Facial Plastic and Reconstructive
    Surgery
1101 Vermont Avenue, Suite 304, Washington, D.C. 20005
202/842-4500

American Society of Plastic and Reconstructive Surgeons
233 North Michigan Avenue, Suite 1900, Chicago, Illinois
    60601
312/856-1834

A support group for people with alopecia areata:

National Alopecia Areata Foundation
P.O. Box 5027, Mill Valley, California 94941
415/383-3444

A support group for men who are bald:

Bald-Headed Men of America
4006 Arendall Avenue, Morehead City, North Carolina
28557

Index

Hamburg, Richard, 81
Hats, 33–34
  after hair transplants, 92
Head standing, 49
Health food store products, 48,
  49, 51
Heart disease, 84
Heat treatments, 49
Helsinki formula, 52–55
  discovery of, 52–53
  effectiveness of, 55
  of Hair Again, Ltd., 54–55
  testing of, 52, 53–54
Helsinki Formula, The (brand),
  53–54
Herbal cures, 49
Heredity
  abnormalities due to, 42
  as factor in pattern baldness,
    20–22, 29
  nature of hair follicles and,
    24
Hix, Charles, 172, 175
Holland, Jimmie, 150
House of Louis Feder, 117,
  125, 127, 128, 130, 153

Implants, synthetic fiber, 102–
  103
Imre, Edith, 153–55
Infections, 42
  hair grafts and, 91
Institute for Loss of Hair, 153,
  154
Iodine, 48

Jacobs, Elliot, 81, 97, 107–8,
  110
Joseph Fleischer (company),
  130–31
Juri flaps, 99

Kahn, Melvin, 69
Kaplan, Ben Z., 121, 122, 124,
  127

Kassimir, Joel J., 67–68, 81, 90,
  100
Kaufman, Theodor, 106–7
Kelp, 48
Krakoff, Lawrence R., 69

Lanugo hair, 24
Lederle Labs, 72
Lederman, Hal Z., 53–54
Lefkovits, Albert, 59, 165, 168
Length of hair, 172–73
Levine, Donald, 81, 96
Loniten (minoxidil)
  See Minoxidil
Looking Good: A Guide for
  Men (Hix), 172, 175

Male pattern baldness (MPB)
  See Pattern baldness
Mann, Maurice, 54–55, 104–6,
  108
Massage, scalp, 48
Mayer, Toby G., 81
Medical insurance
  for hair extensions, 141
  for hairpieces, 128
  for hair transplants, 93
  for wigs, 129, 155
MEDI-PRO, 168
Men's Hair (Roberson), 167
Mervis, Phyllis, 151
Messner, Carolyn, 151
Microplugs, 83
Miller, Evan, 134, 137, 139,
  140
Minoxidil, 12–13, 15, 29, 41,
  60–72
  business community interest
    in, 64–65
  current use of, 65–67
  effect on hair follicles, 61
  expert opinions of, 67–71
  FDA approval and, 65
  patient opinions of, 71–72

Minoxidil *(cont.)*
  testing of, 62–64, 67–72
  use of hair transplants, 89–
    90
Moles, 43
Mustaches, 24, 175

Nida, Edward R., 51

Oily hair, 166, 169
Olsen, Elise, 69
Olsen, Ray, 170, 173, 175
Oncologists, 147
Oral contraceptives, 29, 35, 42
Orentreich, Norman, 48, 57–
    58, 79, 80, 81

Pantron 1, 53–54
Parting hair, 170–72
Pattern baldness, 19–22, 25–
    30
  age as factor in, 20, 27–28,
    29
  androgens as cause of, 20,
    21–22, 27, 29
  hereditary factors in, 20–22,
    29
  prevalence of, 20–21
  remedies for
    See Remedies, nonsurgical;
      Surgical remedies
  sequence of hair loss in, 25–
    26, 28
  among women, 20, 28–30
Pearlstein, Hillard, 70, 81
Permanent waves, 36, 173–74
Physical stress, 31–32, 34
Physicians
  hair loss consultation, 33,
    36–37, 44
  hair restorers and, 51, 57–59
  hair transplants and
    See Hair transplants
    See also Surgical remedies
Pilo-Genic Research

Associates, Inc., 55–57
Placebo, 63
Plugs, 82–83
  See also Hair transplants
Policar, Joseph, 66
Polysorbate
  See Helsinki formula
Preauricular flaps, 99
Pregnancy, 35
Price, Vera, 165–66, 167, 168
Progesterone, 57–58, 59
Prostaglandin, 72
Protein
  in conditioners and rinses,
    166–68
  in diet, 34, 48
PUVA (psoralen ultraviolet
    light), 40–41

Radiation therapy
  hair loss as sing of illness,
    149–51
  hair loss due to, 147
  permanent hair loss from,
    154
  regrowth of hair after, 147
Reduction of scalp, 94–96
Reed, Michael Lorin, 68–69
Regaine Topical Solution, 65
Remedies, nonsurgical, 47–73
  Aldactone (spironolactone),
    58
  biotin products, 55–57
  brushing, 48–49
  folk, 49
  hair restorers, 49–51
  heat treatments, 49
  Helsinki formula, 52–55
  minoxidil
    See Minoxidil
  Progesterone, 57–58, 59
  prostaglandin, 72
  slant boards and head
    standing, 49
  special foods, 48

About the Author

MARY-ELLEN SIEGEL FIRST LEARNED HOW DEVASTATING HAIR loss can be when she was three years old. Because her hair had fallen out following an illness, she was one day mistaken for a boy.

Since then she has raised three children, graduated summa cum laude from the City University of New York, earned a master's degree in social work from Columbia University, and has written six books. She and her husband have six grandsons ranging from one to eight years old, who will learn they don't have to be bald, if they don't want to be. All they have to do is read this book.

Ms. Siegel is a senior teaching associate in the Department of Community Medicine (Social Work), Mount Sinai School of Medicine, in New York City. She is a social worker/therapist in private practice.